WN17 W1

**WORLD HEALTH ORGANIZATION
BASIC RADIOLOGICAL SYSTEM**

**MANUAL OF RADIOGRAPHIC INTERPRETATION
FOR GENERAL PRACTITIONERS**

World Health Organization Basic Radiological System

# Manual of Radiographic Interpretation for General Practitioners

by

**P.E.S. Palmer**
University of California, Davis,
California, United States of America

**W.P. Cockshott**
MacMaster University, Hamilton, Canada

**V. Hegedüs**
Glostrup Hospital, Glostrup, Denmark

**E. Samuel**
University of Edinburgh, Scotland

**WORLD HEALTH ORGANIZATION**
**GENEVA**
**1985**

Reprinted 1986, 1987

ISBN 92 4 154177 6

PRINTED IN SWITZERLAND
83/5935 – 86/6664 – 12 000
87/7362 – Atar – 8000 (R)

# CONTENTS

# INTRODUCTION

## The World Health Organization Basic Radiological System—BRS

The concept of primary health care cannot be successfully implemented without the support of diagnostic services. Such services must include facilities for diagnostic radiology. Accordingly, a few years ago WHO initiated the development of a "Basic Radiological System" (BRS) to provide better radiological coverage for populations at present underserved.

Apart from their general inadequacy, the existing radiodiagnostic facilities in developing countries seldom meet the real needs of the majority of the population. Eighty per cent of all X-ray examinations are essentially simple procedures: in the developing world the percentage is nearer ninety, given the lack of sophisticated equipment and the paucity of highly specialized personnel. Thus, a well-structured radiological network should operate at three levels. Health centres and rural hospitals should be equipped to manage only basic radiological examinations, such as those of the chest, abdomen, and skeleton, and simple (nonfluoroscopic) contrast examinations. Radiologists and radiographers would not be required, except for referral, to solve difficult problems. The general hospital—the next level—should provide general-purpose radiological examinations, adding a fluoroscopy unit as well as the unmodified BRS equipment: a radiologist and several radiographers would be required. Finally, a specialized and comprehensive radiological service should be available at specialized centres and university hospitals.

Thus, the Basic Radiological System has been devised for primary health care units, located at peripheral hospitals, small polyclinics, health centres, etc., to look after a population of 25 000–200 000. Such a system needs not only a suitable X-ray installation (now available as the WHO–BRS unit) but training for the operators and general medical practitioners who will have recourse to equipment.

Because all of the most common conditions in which there are radiographic abnormalities can be demonstrated by the WHO–BRS, the selection of material for inclusion in the present manual proved to be a formidable task. The WHO–BRS Advisory Group—all radiologists with wide experience both in the industrialized and in the developing world—was responsible for preparing this diagnostic manual.[1] In so doing, it has tried to produce a book that will help the doctor who does not have ready access to a radiologist, and who must make the right decisions without delay.

Primary decision-making does not always include an immediate X-ray examination: in many cases treatment must immediately follow clinical assessment. The X-ray examination may come much later, or not at all. But the diagnostic X-ray film may help to decide whether the patient can continue treatment at the primary centre or whether he[2] must be referred to a larger hospital—and when the transfer should take place.

---

[1] The members of the WHO–BRS Advisory Group are as follows: Mr E. Borg, Sana'a, Yemen; Professor W. P. Cockshott, MacMaster University, Hamilton, Ontario, Canada; Dr V. Hegedūs, University of Copenhagen, Glostrup, Denmark; Dr T. Holm, University Hospital, Lund, Sweden; Dr J. J. Lyimo, Kilimanjaro Christian Medical Centre, Moshi, United Republic of Tanzania; Professor P. E. S. Palmer, University of California, Davis, CA, United States of America; and Professor E. Samuel, Edinburgh, Scotland.

The Group was also responsible for compiling the technical specifications of the BRS, as well as a *Manual of Radiographic Technique* and a *Manual of Darkroom Technique*, both to be published by WHO.

[2] For the sake of convenience, throughout this manual the masculine gender has been used for pronouns referring to "the patient".

Not every disease or injury can be described in such a small manual; moreover, conditions of frequent occurrence in one geographical area may be rare in another. The manual concentrates on diagnostic problems that are common universally; many of these can be successfully managed at the primary care level.

Ideally, special courses in diagnostic radiology, lasting a few weeks and linked to this manual, should be part of the training of all general practitioners. The need for consultation would have to be stressed, and in this connexion a regional network linking general practitioners, radiologists and other specialists would have to be built up. The isolated doctor with a BRS unit will face many difficult diagnostic problems and must recognize the need for help as an essential part of patient care.

The BRS Advisory Group would greatly welcome any comments or suggestions regarding this manual from the general practitioners who use it and the specialists to whom problem cases are referred. Such advice and guidance would be of considerable value in the revision of any subsequent edition. The more comments that are received, the more the manual—and, ultimately, patient care—can be improved. Such observations should be sent to: Chief Medical Officer, Radiation Medicine, World Health Organization, 1211 Geneva 27, Switzerland.

Finally, it may be noted that the WHO–BRS unit produces such high-quality radiographs that its use should not be limited to the developing world. It may well provide a very important solution to the escalating cost of health care in even the most advanced countries.

ALTHOUGH THIS MANUAL IS ADDRESSED TO PHYSICIANS, IT PRESENTS IN THE FOLLOWING SECTION (YELLOW PAGES) INSTRUCTIONS PRIMARILY INTENDED FOR BRS OPERATORS. THIS MATERIAL HAS BEEN INCLUDED BECAUSE **IT IS THE MEDICAL PRACTITIONER'S RESPONSIBILITY TO TRAIN THE BRS OPERATOR TO DEAL WITH ANY EMERGENCY IN THE X-RAY DEPARTMENT.**

PLEASE READ THESE YELLOW PAGES AS SOON AS YOU CAN
AND
BEFORE YOU REQUEST ANY X-RAY EXAMINATION NEEDING
AN INJECTION OF A RADIOLOGICAL CONTRAST DRUG

- The yellow pages contain EMERGENCY instructions.
- They tell you how to treat any drug reactions that may occur.
- It is the duty of every health care practitioner to train all BRS operators to recognize and manage any patient who has an adverse reaction to a drug.

(The same pages are included in the BRS *Manual of Radiographic Technique.*)

# RADIATION PROTECTION
# THE RISK OF HARM FROM X-RAYS

X-RAYS ARE ONLY DANGEROUS IF YOU ARE CARELESS.

*Care means adhering to the following rules:*

— Stand behind the control panel when the X-ray exposure is made.
— Make sure that lead aprons and lead gloves are worn if the patient needs to be held.
— If possible, do not allow anyone else in the X-ray room. If other persons must be present, keep them behind the control panel when the exposure is made.
— When supplied, wear your film badge always. Have it checked regularly.
— Never take an X-ray unless ordered by a DOCTOR or other qualified medical person.

X-rays may cause harm. You cannot FEEL OR SEE THEM: you may not know you are in the X-ray beam, but REPEATED exposure to X-rays, even those that are scattered off the patient or the X-ray equipment, and even in small doses, can cause permanent damage to the health of the X-ray operator or anyone else. Remember again, it is not only the direct beam of X-rays that may be harmful, but also the scattered rays.

You must NEVER make an X-ray exposure when you are anywhere near the X-ray tube: you must always be behind the control panel. There you are safe.

You must NOT allow anyone except the patient to be in the X-ray room, unless the patient needs to be supported or a child needs to be held. When that is necessary, the parent or friend must wear a lead apron and lead gloves whenever he or she is near the patient while the X-ray is being taken. Do NOT let a nurse or any other member of the hospital staff hold a patient while an exposure is being made.

The risk for patients being X-rayed is very low because they are exposed to X-rays infrequently, and because only a small part of the body is exposed for each picture. But try to get all the details right the first time so that there is no need for a second exposure.

The greatest risk from X-rays is for the operator and the doctor and nurses, who may be exposed repeatedly over the years while they are working. But there is no danger if YOU and THEY ARE CAREFUL.

X-RAYS MAY CAUSE HARM EVEN THOUGH YOU DO NOT SEE OR FEEL THEM.

# REACTIONS TO INTRAVENOUS DRUGS USED FOR UROGRAPHY

Contrast drugs are used for urography (the kidneys, ureters, and bladder). THESE DRUGS MUST ONLY BE INJECTED BY A DOCTOR OR WITH THE DOCTOR'S PERMISSION. There must be a doctor in the hospital and immediately available whenever these drugs are given, until the X-ray examination is finished (although, provided the doctor can be reached quickly, he or she need not actually be in the X-ray room).

The drugs used in urography must be injected into a vein: they make it possible to see the kidneys, ureters, and bladder, which are normally invisible on radiographs. All these drugs are complex iodine compounds; they can produce reactions in the patient that range from mild to very serious, and can—in rare instances—even cause death.

Reactions to drugs can occur at the beginning of the injection, or shortly afterwards, or may even be delayed for 20–40 minutes after the injection. The reaction does not depend on how much of the drug has been injected; a small amount may cause as much reaction as a large amount. There is no way to test the patient before the injection.

Mild reactions are not uncommon (do not be misled by an epileptic fit), but very serious reactions are fortunately rare. Anyone may react: drug reactions are not specifically associated with any other form of allergy, although patients such as asthmatics may react more readily than those who have no history of allergy. No one can be sure that he will not react. If patients have had this type of X-ray examination before and have reacted, try to find out which drug was used. They are less likely to react a second time if a different contrast drug is injected. But when patients have reacted previously you must be ready for another reaction.

APPROPRIATE TREATMENT MUST ALWAYS BE READILY AVAILABLE (ANTIHISTAMINES, STEROIDS, EPINEPHRINE, ATROPINE, AND INTRAVENOUS SALINE) BEFORE CONTRAST DRUGS ARE INJECTED. SPECIAL CARE IS NECESSARY WITH THE CONTRAST DRUGS USED FOR CHOLANGIOGRAPHY.

**TWO BASIC RULES:**

(1) MAKE SURE THAT THE DRUGS ARE AVAILABLE FOR TREATMENT IMMEDIATELY **BEFORE** THE CONTRAST INJECTION.

(2) WHEN CONTRAST DRUGS HAVE BEEN INJECTED INTRAVENOUSLY, NEVER LEAVE THE PATIENT UNATTENDED UNTIL THE EXAMINATION IS COMPLETED AND THE PATIENT FEELS WELL. NO PATIENT WILL HAVE A SERIOUS REACTION AFTER 60 MINUTES.

---

**BE WISE:**
IF THE PATIENT HAS A HISTORY OF REACTION TO PREVIOUS CONTRAST INJECTIONS OR A HISTORY OF SEVERE ALLERGY, REFER HIM TO A MAJOR HOSPITAL FOR THE EXAMINATION.

MAKE SURE THAT YOU HAVE INTRAVENOUS ATROPINE, ANTIHISTAMINE, INTRAVENOUS EPINEPHRINE, AND SOLUBLE STEROIDS AVAILABLE WITH SYRINGES IN OR CLOSE TO THE X-RAY ROOM WHENEVER CONTRAST DRUGS ARE BEING GIVEN.

---

## MILD CONTRAST REACTIONS

The patient will complain of a sensation of heat and pressure in the abdomen, may sneeze, develop urticaria (raised patches on the skin), feel nauseous, and become restless.

### Treatment

Reassure the patient. Tell him not to worry, the reaction will soon go away. Loosen the patient's clothing if it is tight. Tell the patient to take deep breaths in and out and to relax.

Stay with the patient and watch carefully until symptoms diminish. If the reaction does not improve in a few moments, send for a doctor or nurse.

## STRONGER CONTRAST REACTIONS

The patient may vomit, become very short of breath (dyspnoea) and the skin may be pale. He may start to sweat and be very restless. The pulse may be rapid.

### Treatment

Keep calm and reassure the patient.

Raise the patient's head and shoulders if he is short of breath.

If vomiting occurs, turn the patient's head to one side to prevent aspiration of vomit.

If there are signs of collapse (pale skin, sweating, rapid pulse) raise the patient's feet and lower the head (if this is possible on the X-ray table). More important, KEEP THE PATIENT LYING DOWN.

Stay with the patient all the time.

Send for qualified help if symptoms do not improve very quickly (after a few minutes).

## SEVERE CONTRAST REACTIONS

Pale skin, sweating, very shallow breathing, rapid and very weak pulse. Loss of consciousness, cardiac arrest.

SEVERE CONTRAST REACTIONS ARE AN EMERGENCY SITUATION. YOU MUST ACT QUICKLY.

- Call for the doctor and nurse.
- Keep the patient warm and start artificial respiration if the patient stops breathing.
- If oxygen is available, give it to the patient if breathing is difficult. Make sure the airway is open.
- When the doctor and nurse arrive, tell them where the emergency drugs are kept.

**Physician's response**

Check the general condition of the patient:

— Is the patient breathing?
— Is there a good airway?
— Is the heart beating?

If not, start cardiopulmonary resuscitation: restore the airway if necessary (see page 19 et seq.).

CHECK THE PULSE

If **SLOW**:

- Give intravenous atropine—0.01mg for an adult.
- ↓ Start an intravenous saline infusion.
- ↓ Continue intravenous saline → Return to ward as soon as possible.

If very **RAPID**:

- Inject epinephrine, 1:1000, intravenously—up to 1 ml.
- ↓ Start an intravenous saline infusion.
- ↓ Repeat epinephrine, 1:1000, if necessary—not more than 1 ml.
- ↓ Inject 50 mg dexamethasone intravenously.
- ↓ Return to ward as soon as possible.

# FIRST AID AND PATIENT CARE
# FOR THE BRS OPERATOR

## INTRODUCTION

(1) Remember

— You are responsible for the patient in the X-ray department.

(2) You must recognize when the patient's condition is getting worse and

— Call immediately for the nurse or doctor (or both).
— Until help is available, you must know what to do and what NOT to do, and you must know how to help the nurse and doctor when they arrive.
— Always work in a calm and quiet way and always reassure the patient. Even ordinary patients who are not very sick may feel apprehensive in an X-ray room. Children may be very frightened. There is no need for this, because they are in no danger, but they are in strange surroundings and need to be reassured.

## LOOKING AFTER THE PATIENT

— Seriously ill patients must be kept lying down, unless they are very short of breath and are more comfortable sitting up.

— If the patient is vomiting, turn him on to his side to keep the throat clear so that he can breathe. Do not move seriously injured patients, but turn their head only.

— Do not move accident patients more than is absolutely necessary. If you must move them, be careful not to make their injuries worse.

> READ THESE INSTRUCTIONS.
>
> PRACTISE ARTIFICIAL RESPIRATION.
>
> PRACTISE MOVING THE PATIENT.

— Whenever the patient has had a serious accident, assume that there is internal injury to the brain, chest, spine, or abdomen. Be extra careful and gentle.

— Do not let patients get cold. Keep them covered and warm. Try to keep the door shut if it is cold outside the X-ray room.

## PRIORITIES
— Is the patient breathing?
— Is the patient conscious?
— Is the patient bleeding?

DO NOT X-RAY A SERIOUSLY ILL OR SEVERELY INJURED PATIENT ALONE. ALWAYS HAVE QUALIFIED HELP WITH YOU. NEVER LEAVE A SERIOUSLY ILL OR INJURED PATIENT UNWATCHED WHILE YOU ARE DEVELOPING THE FILMS OR HAVE TO LEAVE THE X-RAY ROOM FOR ANY OTHER REASON. GET A NURSE, ORDERLY, OR SOME OTHER TRAINED PERSON TO STAY WITH THE PATIENT ALL THE TIME.

## WHAT TO DO IF THE PATIENT STOPS BREATHING

— Always check to make sure that an unconscious person is breathing; do this often. He may stop breathing quietly without any cough or other noise. This can happen quite suddenly without warning.

— If the patient stops breathing, make sure that the air passage is open. Gently tilt the head backwards and lift the chin upwards (see next page). If the patient is wearing dentures, remove them.

— Close the nose with your fingers, and hold the jaw up with the other hand. Give mouth-to-nose or mouth-to-mouth artificial respiration at the rate of 12–15 breaths per minute (see pages 19–22).

— When the patient starts breathing, and if he is not too badly injured, turn him into the lateral safety position (see pages 24–25).

### IMPORTANT RULES

(1) TALK TO THE PATIENT TO SEE IF HE IS CONSCIOUS BEFORE YOU GIVE RESPIRATION.

(2) CHECK THE MOUTH AND THE THROAT TO MAKE SURE THAT NOTHING IS BLOCKING THE AIRWAY (FOOD, DIRT, VOMIT). CLEAN THE MOUTH AND THROAT IF NECESSARY.

(3) IF THE PATIENT IS NOT BREATHING, START ARTIFICIAL RESPIRATION WHEN YOU HAVE CLEANED THE AIRWAY.

(4) IF YOU CANNOT CLEAN THE AIRWAY COMPLETELY, TURN THE PATIENT'S HEAD TO ONE SIDE, WHICH IS USUALLY ENOUGH TO ALLOW AIR TO ENTER THE CHEST.

(5) CALL FOR HELP—FOR A NURSE AND DOCTOR—IMMEDIATELY.

(6) LOOSEN THE PATIENT'S TIGHT CLOTHING.

# ARTIFICIAL RESPIRATION

## Clearing the Airway

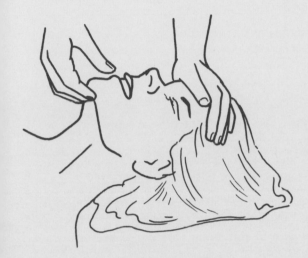

The muscles of an unconscious person are completely relaxed. The tongue, being a muscle that is fixed to the lower jaw, will fall back and close the throat if the patient is kept lying on his back.

To remove this obstruction:

(1) Kneel next to the patient's head.

(2) Put one of your hands on to the patient's forehead and the other under the patient's chin.

(3) Lift the lower jaw of the patient upwards and tilt the head backwards until the chin is higher than the nose.

(4) This gives a free air-passage by lifting the tongue away from the back wall of the throat.

(5) Keeping the head in this position, listen and look to check whether breathing has started again.

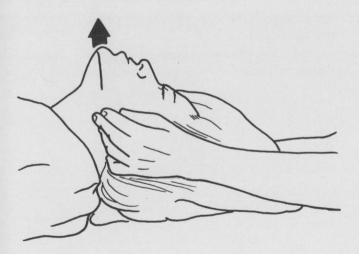

If breathing starts, turn the patient to the lateral safety position (see pages 24–25).

If there is no breathing continue with artificial respiration.

You can revive a patient by blowing air through his nose into his lungs, or through his mouth into his lungs. For children (see page 22), this must be done very carefully.

You must practise this and know exactly how to carry out artificial respiration. You must also REMEMBER TO CLEAR THE AIRWAY before you start (see previous page).

## Mouth-to-Nose Respiration

head tilt—neck lift

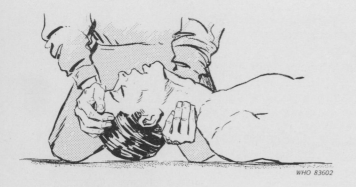

WHO 83602

Tilt the head so that the chin is higher than the nose.

Close the mouth of the patient by pushing the lower lip upwards with your thumb.

Open your mouth wide, take a deep breath and place your mouth firmly around the patient's nose.

Blow air into the patient's lungs. Take your mouth away from the nose. This must be done every 5 seconds until regular breathing is restored.

Lift your head, look at the patient's chest to see whether the ribs are moving. If not, take another deep breath and blow once more through the patient's nose.

Continue until the patient starts breathing without help.

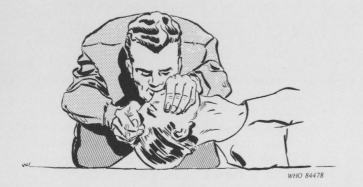

WHO 84478

BLOW AIR INTO THE PATIENT'S LUNGS EVERY 5 SECONDS UNTIL REGULAR BREATHING STARTS AGAIN OR UNTIL A QUALIFIED PERSON TELLS YOU TO STOP.

## Mouth-to-Mouth Respiration

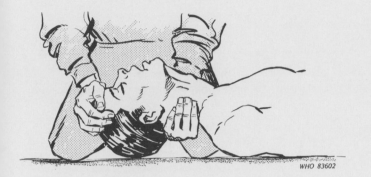

WHO 83602

Put one hand under the patient's neck and the other hand on the patient's forehead.

Tilt the patient's head backwards until the chin is higher than the nose, lifting the neck as you push the forehead down.

Sometimes the patient will then start breathing. Watch the chest carefully in case this has happened.

If the patient has not started breathing, then you must start artificial respiration immediately.

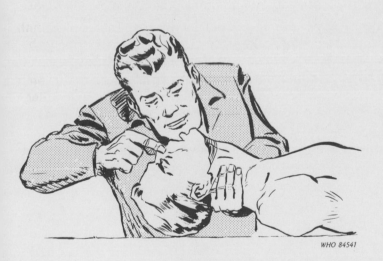

WHO 84541

Keep the head extended by lifting the neck; pinch the patient's nose with your thumb and forefinger.

Take a deep breath and place your mouth firmly over the patient's mouth.

Blow air into the patient's lungs. Take your mouth away from the patient and your thumb and forefinger away from the nose. (Keep the other hand under the neck.)

Look at the ribs. The chest will collapse when you stop blowing air and this will tell you that you have been successful in getting air into the lungs. If the ribs do not move inward, check the airway to make sure that it is not blocked and lift the hand under the neck to make sure that it is sufficiently extended.

If the patient does not start breathing again, take another deep breath and start the routine once more.

**Artificial Respiration for Babies**

When you have to help a baby to start breathing, you lift the head back gently, but not as far as for an adult or a large child.

A baby's face is so small that you may not be able to close the nose and blow through the mouth alone. You may have to blow through both at the same time.

Put your mouth firmly around the baby's *mouth and nose* and blow gently every 3 seconds (about 20 breaths per minute). Watch to see how the chest moves. Small puffs of air will probably be enough for infants.

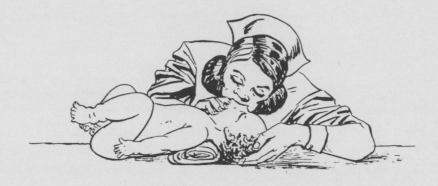

WHENEVER A PERSON NEEDS ARTIFICIAL RESPIRATION, YOU MUST CALL FOR QUALIFIED HELP **BUT YOU MUST NOT WAIT. YOU MUST START ARTIFICIAL RESPIRATION AT ONCE.**

## WHEN THE HEART STOPS

BEGIN AT ONCE:

CHECK THE CAROTID (NECK) ARTERY FOR THE PULSE. IF THIS IS ABSENT:

    (1) Turn the patient on to his BACK—supine.

    (2) Open the air passages (use an artificial airway and bag and mask with oxygen if available and you are trained to do so).

    (3) Place both hands flat on the lower end of the sternum (one hand above the other).

    (4) Keep your arms straight above the sternum. Press straight down.

    80 COMPRESSIONS PER MINUTE (ADULTS) with full relaxation in between each compression.

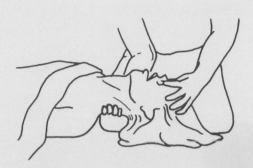

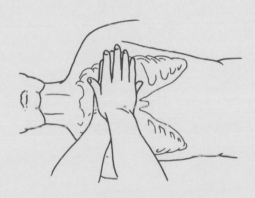

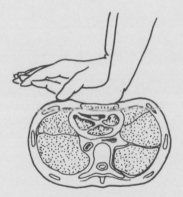

    (5) INFANTS NEED 100 COMPRESSIONS PER MINUTE: use fingertips to compress. DO NOT PRESS TOO HARD on a baby or small child.

    Ventilate (with air or oxygen) after every 5 cardiac compressions (more in children).

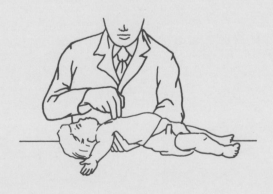

## LATERAL SAFETY POSITION

When a person is unconscious his muscles are completely relaxed. The tongue (which is also a muscle and is fixed to the lower jaw) falls backwards if the patient is lying on his back and it will block the throat and prevent breathing.

To open the airway, turn patient on to his side, tilting him forward as shown in the drawings. In this position the tongue cannot fall back and any blood, phlegm, or vomit can run out of the mouth without blocking the airway.

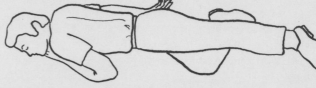

This is how you move the patient.

(1) Kneel down on the side to which you are going to turn the patient.

(2) Stretch the patient's nearer arm along his body and put the palm of the patient's hand under the buttocks.

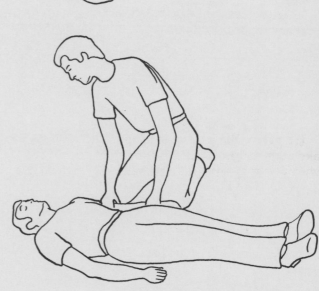

(3) Bend the leg of the patient which is nearer to you at the hip and the knee, putting your hand under the knee and lifting. At the same time, fold the patients' other arm (the one further away from you) across the chest so that the fingers are close to the side of the patient's head which is nearer to you.

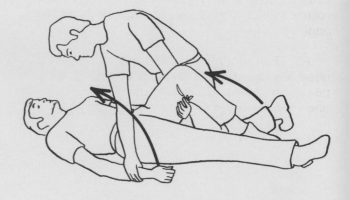

(4) Put one of your hands on the shoulder of the patient which is further away from you and the other on the hip which is further away from you.

Turn the patient toward you, pulling steadily and rolling the patient over the arm which is nearer to you.

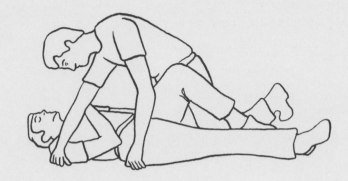

(5) When the patient is lying on his side (facing you), take your hand off his shoulder and support the head while you move the rest of the body towards you.

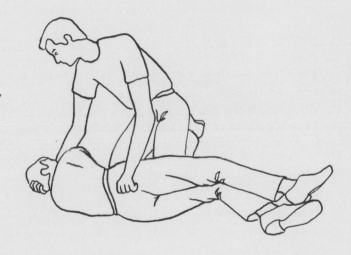

(6) When the patient is lying on his stomach, pull the lower arm (the arm over which the patient rolled) and let it lie alongside. Put the other hand under the cheek.

(7) Then move the patient's head so that it is tilted backwards with the neck extended, to maintain the free air-passage. Adjust the patient's legs, one over the other as shown in the drawing.

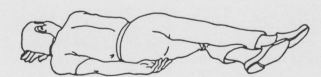

**NOTES**

# CHEST X-RAYS

# CHEST X-RAYS

## CHOICE OF VIEWS

*A postero-anterior (PA) (or antero-posterior (AP) for children) view* is usually sufficient. If an abnormality is seen, a lateral view should then be added. However, the lateral view should only be taken when the PA view has been inspected.

*Which lateral view?* Take the LEFT lateral view unless all the clinical symptoms and signs are on the right, in which case take the right lateral view.

*Erect or supine?* Whenever possible take the chest X-ray in the erect or sitting position, because many intrathoracic conditions (e.g., pleural fluid, pneumothorax, heart size, mediastinal width) are difficult to assess when the film is taken with the patient lying down.

*Apical (lordotic) views* are used ONLY when the PA film shows a possible abnormality in the apical area of either lung. The additional views should only be taken AFTER THE ROUTINE FILM HAS BEEN VIEWED, and when there is difficulty in interpreting an apical lesion.

*Decubitus views* are taken when there is strong clinical suspicion of pleural fluid but none can be seen on the PA or lateral films. The decubitus views are taken ONLY after the routine PA and lateral projections have been viewed.

*Rib oblique films* are taken ONLY for RIB abnormalities (e.g., local swelling) or when there is localized, unexplained pain in the chest, and only after the routine films have been reviewed. Even with good oblique films, rib fractures may not be seen.

*An "expiratory" film* is a chest X-ray taken in the PA or AP position with the patient in full expiration, breathing out. It is only taken when routine films fail to reveal a clinically suspected pneumothorax or an inhaled foreign body.

# CHEST INTERPRETATION

Follow a systematic method in inspecting the chest radiograph.

(1) (a) Check that the film is correctly centred, and is taken in full inspiration (page 32). A film taken in expiration can cause confusion: it may simulate disease, e.g., pulmonary congestion, cardio-megaly, or a wide mediastinum; exclude shadows due to hair, clothing, or skin lesions.

(b) Check that the exposure is correct (a finger held behind the "black area" of the film should be just visible when correct density has been achieved). An underexposed (pale) film must be inter-preted with caution; the lung appearance may suggest pulmonary oedema or consolidation. Over-exposure (a black film) may suggest emphysema.

(2) Check that the bony skeleton (ribs, clavicles, scapula, etc.) is normal.

(3) Check that the diaphragm is normal in position; the right side of the diaphragm is usually 2.5 cm higher than the left (identified in the lateral view by the gas bubble in the stomach or colon beneath it, see page 30). Check costophrenic angles in both PA and lateral films.

(4) Check the superior mediastinum for widening, or the presence of abnormal masses, and identify the trachea.

(5) Check the heart and great vessels for abnormalities. The cardiac diameter in adults (erect film) should be less than half the width of the chest.

(6) (a) All the markings in normal lungs are vascular. Check that they are normal in size and pattern ("lung pattern").

(b) The hilar shadows should show individual vessels representing the pulmonary arteries and large veins. It may be difficult to see other pulmonary veins. The left hilum is normally higher than the right.

(c) Remember that the pulmonary and cardiac systems are intimately related and that pulmonary changes (e.g., oedema) may be secondary to cardiac changes.

A normal chest X-ray does NOT exclude developing pulmonary disease, especially in children; abnormali-ties visible on a chest X-ray may take longer to develop than the clinical abnormalities.

Follow-up films. The clinical condition of the patient must decide when follow-up films need to be taken; if clinical progress is satisfactory, further films may not be necessary. If the clinical condition requires further films, a single PA film is usually sufficient.

## Normal Chest, PA View

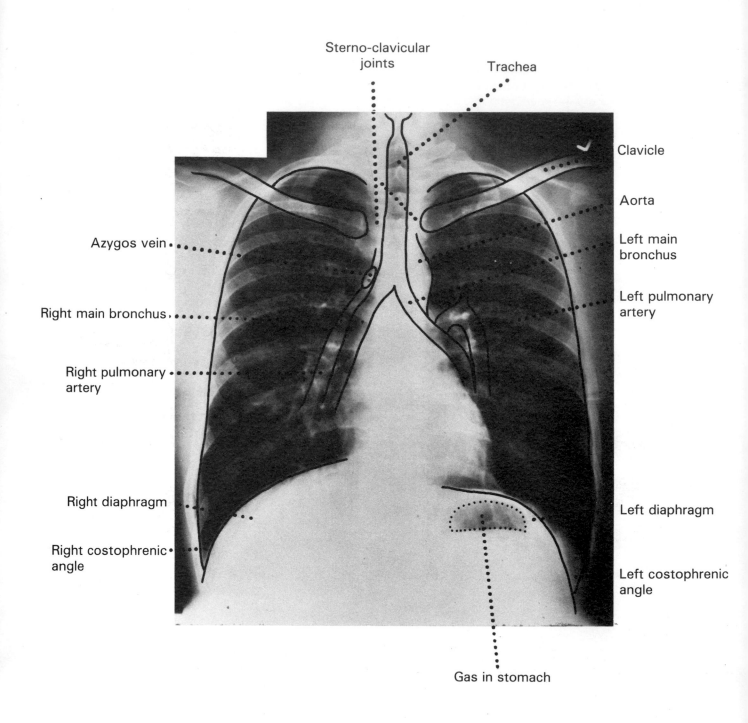

Sterno-clavicular joints

Trachea

Clavicle

Azygos vein

Aorta

Left main bronchus

Right main bronchus

Left pulmonary artery

Right pulmonary artery

Right diaphragm

Left diaphragm

Right costophrenic angle

Left costophrenic angle

Gas in stomach

## Normal Chest, Lateral View

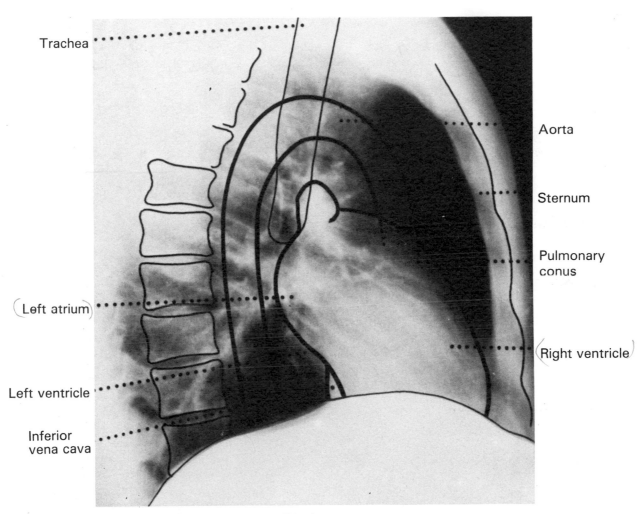

Trachea

Aorta

Sternum

Pulmonary
conus

Left atrium

Right ventricle

Left ventricle

Inferior
vena cava

Diaphragm

## TECHNICAL FAULT MIMICKING DISEASE

Many errors in diagnosis are the result of faulty radiographic technique—especially on chest radiographs. Technical faults may mimic disease.

**Poor Inspiration**

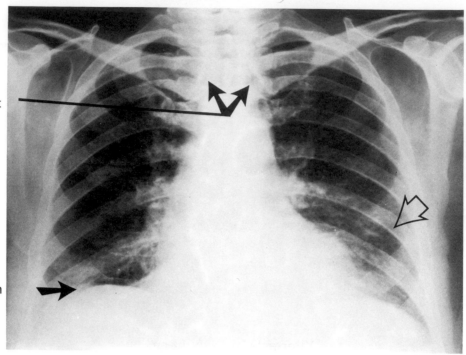

**Unsatisfactory**

Sterno-clavicular joints equidistant from mid-line.

Increased markings in both lower lobes.

High diaphragm (anterior end of 5th rib).

Increased cardiac diameter.

**Full Inspiration**

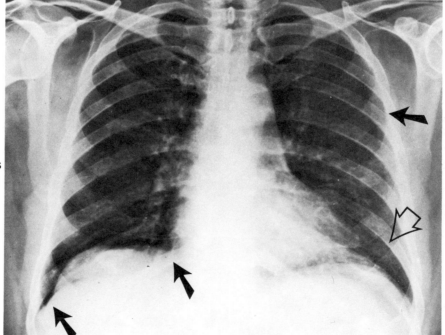

**Satisfactory**

Scapula clear of lung fields.

Diaphragm crosses anterior end of 6th rib.

Normal lung markings in lower lobes.

Costophrenic angle sharp.          Cardiophrenic angle acute.

## Supine Chest

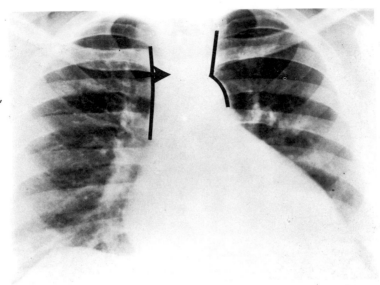

The mediastinum may appear wide, perhaps 10 cm.

Prominent pulmonary vessels, especially in the upper lobes.

The heart appears enlarged. Never diagnose a large heart *or* congestive cardiac failure from a radiograph taken when the patient is supine.

## "Portable" or Ward Film

Patients who are sitting up in bed (*or* who are in the last weeks of pregnancy *or* who have a large liver or ascites) cannot take a full inspiration.

*Poor Inspiration*

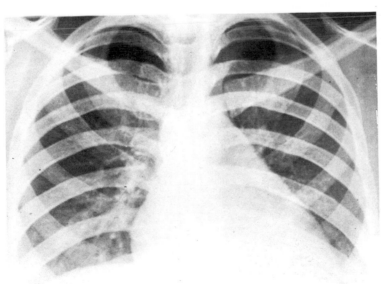

Pulmonary vessels prominent: often crowded at the lung base (may resemble pneumonia).

Heart appears enlarged: left cardiac border may appear flattened.

BAD POSITIONING — INCORRECT EXPOSURE — POOR INSPIRATION — FAILURE TO STOP BREATHING — ALL LEAD TO ERRORS IN INTERPRETATION OF THE RADIOGRAPH.

# PAIN IN CHEST

Chest X-rays are of no help in angina and painful pericarditis.

Not all patients with chest pain have abnormal chest X-rays, but those who present with localized pain in the chest *without* marked coughing may show:

(a) Fractured ribs or other rib abnormalities (history of trauma, page 37).

(b) Pneumothorax (page 39), usually with a history of trauma or sudden pain.

(c) Pleurisy or pleural effusion (page 41).

(d) If aortic dissection or aneurysm is suspected clinically as a cause of pain, a PA film may be helpful. A repeat examination a few hours later may help to show the change. However, do not compare an erect film with a supine film. The supine film can be misleading because the mediastinum often appears widened when supine, even in normal people.

(e) If it is clinically necessary to demonstrate rib pathology or fractures, oblique views should be taken, localized to the area suspected after clinical examination (page 37).

# ACUTE CHEST TRAUMA

Damage to intrathoracic contents may occur with both open and closed chest injuries. The diagnosis of a tension pneumothorax should be made clinically and treatment started without waiting for X-ray examinations.

However, chest X-rays are useful for management and to exclude a non-tension pneumothorax or intrapleural or pulmonary bleeding.

### Pneumothorax (may need decompression)

(1)  Look for the edge of the collapsed lung (where the lung markings stop). A fold of skin can look like a pneumothorax, especially in children or the elderly. Confirm by clinical examination.

(2)  There may be mediastinal and tracheal shift AWAY from the injured side (expiratory films demonstrate this clearly).

(3)  A supine film may appear normal, even when there is a small pneumothorax.

(4)  Subcutaneous emphysema. Air in the soft tissues of the chest wall may spread across the chest, axilla, and neck, and if there is a large quantity it may hide an underlying pneumothorax. (Check to make sure there is no shift of the trachea and mediastinum. Shift can only be due to air *inside* the chest.)

### Internal bleeding

(1)  *Into the pleura.* Look for the white density of a haemothorax (which is not always obvious on a supine film). The heart and trachea may be shifted away from the injured side, and this indicates a large haemorrhage.

(2)  *Into the pericardium* after stab wounds. Look for bleeding into the pericardium, which may be suspected when there is an increase in the cardiac size and the heart shape becomes globular. In the early stages clinical features are more important.

(3)  *Into the mediastinum:*

(a)  If there is widening of the mediastinum check both radial pulses and take the blood pressure in each arm. Look for fractures of the upper ribs.

(b)  Look for progressive increase in size of the mediastinum on sequential films. Remember that the mediastinum always appears wide on a supine chest film and that slight rotation of the patient may exaggerate the width even when the mediastinum is normal. Repeat the AP film, or, better still, if the patient can sit or stand, take an erect film.

## Closed Chest Injuries

### *Fractured ribs*

Normally there is no need to X-ray the chest when rib fractures are suspected, unless there is clinical indication of damage to the lung or pleura. Rib-oblique films will usually be necessary to see the rib fractures.

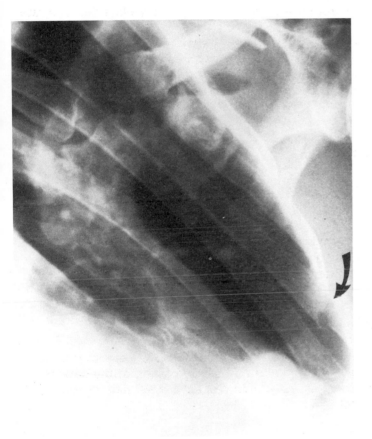

Rib fractures may not be seen on routine chest films.

Fracture near anterior ends of left ribs

Rib-oblique views demonstrate the fractures more clearly than ordinary chest films or lateral views, but even the demonstration of fractures seldom affects treatment.

To search for fractured ribs, look carefully at each rib over its complete length, not only at the site of pain. If necessary, examine the film under a bright light. Fractures are difficult to see if there is no displacement, but look also for pleural fluid in the costophrenic angle, and associated pneumothorax, and any underlying pulmonary collapse.

Callus around the healing fracture or the deformity of an old fracture can resemble a rib abnormality and may even suggest a tumour.

## Closed Chest Injuries *(continued)*

Injuries to the chest wall may be penetrating (open) wounds or closed, when the chest wall is not penetrated.

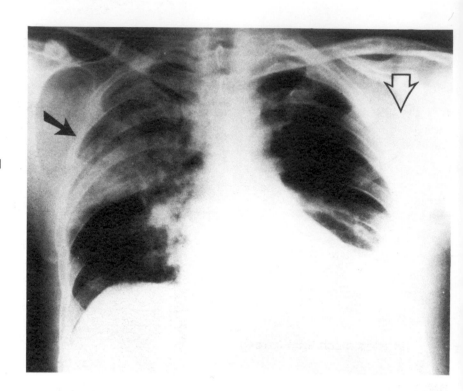

### *Closed injury*

Haematoma in chest wall causing soft-tissue swelling and obscuring rib fractures (seen on the oblique films, hollow arrow).

Violent compression of the chest wall can cause a pulmonary haematoma without causing rib fractures. This may be diffuse and look like consolidation (black arrow), or appear as an ill-defined solitary round shadow.

Haematomas usually resolve in days or weeks unless they become infected (which will be suspected clinically).

## Open Chest Injuries

### *Penetrating injury*

Bullet or stab wounds may cause bleeding along the track, or a pulmonary haematoma, appearing as an area of consolidation.

Air in subcutaneous tissues (subcutaneous emphysema) associated with the bullet wound (hollow arrow).

Traumatic pulmonary haematoma associated with the bullet track.

Bullet lodged in posterior chest wall. It was shown not to be in the lung by the lateral view.

**Penetrating Chest Injuries**
**Subcutaneous Emphysema and Pneumothorax**

*PA view*

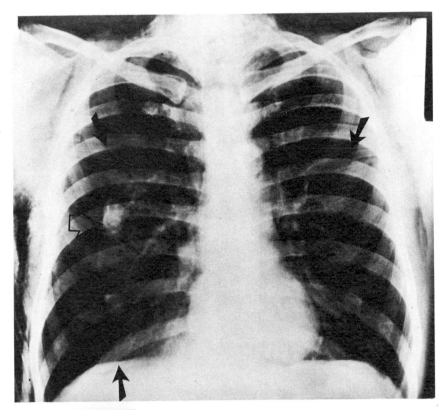

Horizontal black lines indicate air between muscle bundles (arrows).

Edge of partially collapsed right lung (hollow arrow).

Flattened diaphragm (arrow).

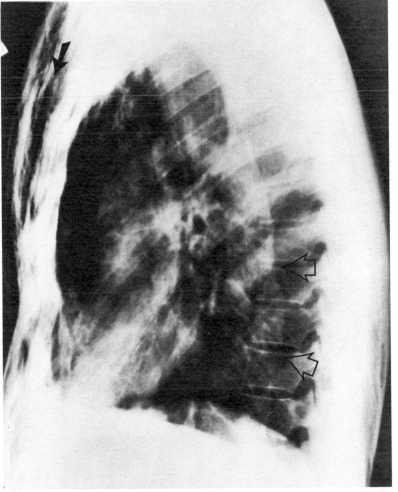

*Right lateral view*

Air in soft tissues (arrow).

Edge of partially collapsed right lung (hollow arrows).

## Inhaled Foreign Body

If any foreign body is inhaled into the bronchi, it may cause partial or complete blockage. When there is partial obstruction, the lung may balloon beyond the blockage, causing obstructive emphysema.

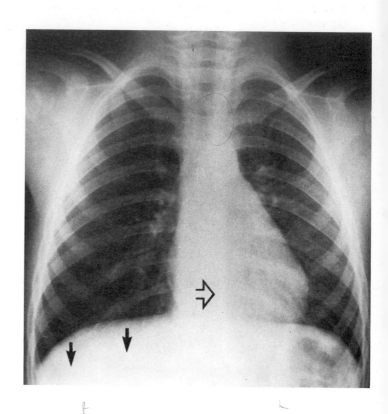

In this patient the foreign body lodged in the right main bronchus, causing over-inflation of the right lung. The mediastinum was then displaced to the left (hollow arrow) and the diaphragm forced downwards. Sometimes a film taken in EXPIRATION will show this more clearly. Remember that the foreign body may not be opaque to X-rays and so may not be visible on the film, but can still cause obstruction.

When the bronchus is *completely blocked,* the segment or lobe of lung distal to the blockage will collapse. Which part of the lung collapses will depend on which bronchus is blocked. In this child, both the right middle lobe and the right lower lobe are collapsed, so the foreign body must be in the bronchus intermedius (below the upper lobe bronchus).

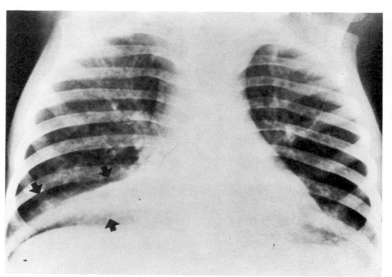

When liquids are inhaled (e.g., soup, liquid paraffin, vomit), there is usually patchy bronchopneumonia. When irritant gases are inhaled (e.g., chlorine), there is usually pulmonary oedema in both lungs.

## PLEURAL EFFUSIONS

(1) A small amount of fluid can be difficult to detect.

(2) It is not possible to differentiate between different types of pleural effusion, e.g., transudate, exudate, blood (haemothorax), pus (empyema), by looking at the X-ray films.

(3) It is very difficult to estimate the amount of fluid radiologically.

(4) It is often difficult to differentiate pleural fluid from pleural thickening or scarring. A decubitus film can be very helpful.

(5) Fluid in the interlobar fissures may resemble a mass (see page 43).

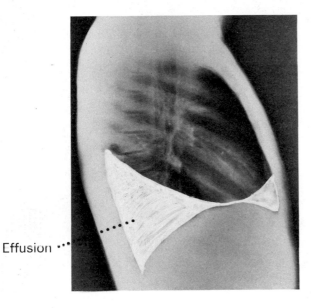

Effusion ·····

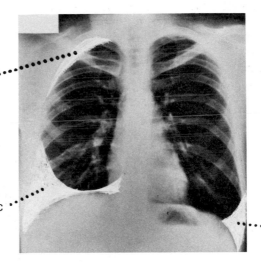

Apical ···········
fluid

Fluid in
costophrenic ·····
angle

·····Small
effusion

*Typical sites for pleural fluid (effusion, pus, or blood)*

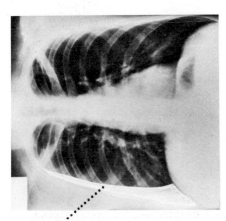

Effusion

If there is any doubt about a pleural effusion, ask for a decubitus view.

This patient is on the right side and the fluid has collected along his lateral chest wall.

When the patient is X-rayed standing or sitting, fluid in the pleural cavity extends upwards along the axillary border in a smooth curve. It may extend over the apex of the lung or into the fissures of the lung (an interlobar effusion, see next page).

*Right pleural effusion* (PA)

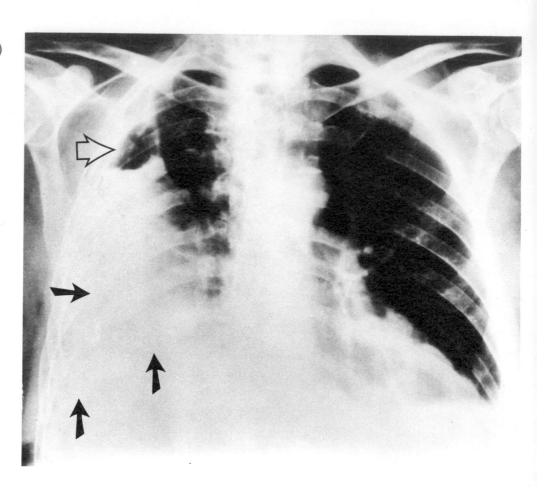

Some of the fluid has been aspirated and air leaked into the pleura, so that there is now air on top of the fluid.

Fluid is causing the density along the axillary border of the chest. Clinically there will be dullness to percussion over this fluid.

The right diaphragm, cardiac border and costophrenic angle have been obscured by the fluid (vertical arrows).

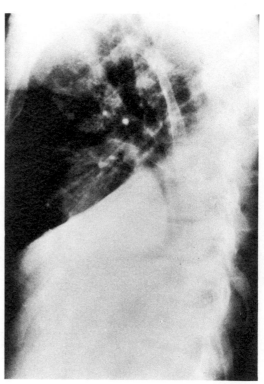

*The lateral view* of a right pleural effusion (different patient). The fluid has obliterated the posterior costophrenic angle and runs up the posterior chest wall. It is not possible to decide whether this is a transudate or exudate, pus or blood. The clinical history and the patient's clinical condition help to make that differential diagnosis. In this patient the "effusion" was blood following injury.

When fluid is BILATERAL, think first of heart failure, renal failure, or occasionally infection (tuberculosis).

## Loculated Effusion

Fluid may locate in any part of the pleural cavity: collections of fluid in the interlobar fissures can look like a mass.

*PA view*

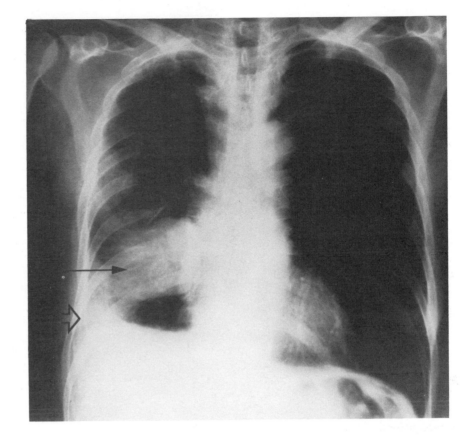

Fluid in lower portion of right major interlobar fissure (black arrow).

Fluid in costophrenic angle of pleural cavity (hollow arrow) obliterating diaphragm.

*Lateral view (same patient)*

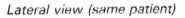

Effusion.

Note the posterior position of the fluid in the fissure (hollow arrow) as well as the fluid in the pleural cavity (black arrow).

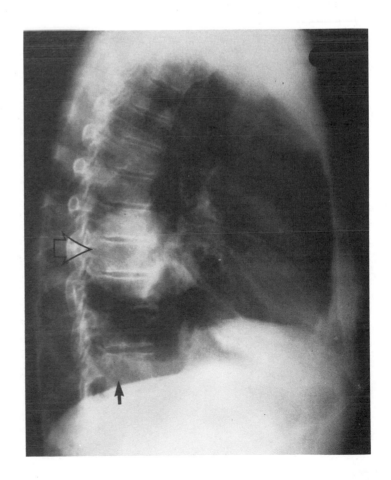

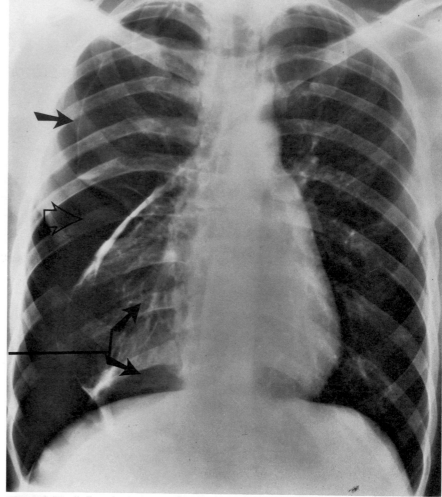

### Pneumothorax

Partially collapsed upper lobe.

When there is air in the pleural cavity, the vascular markings will be absent outside the lung.

The middle and lower lobes are partially collapsed, to a greater extent than the upper lobe.

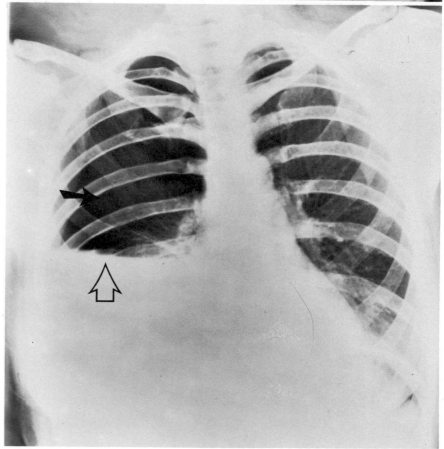

### Hydropneumothorax

The right lung is so collapsed that it is only just visible.

Air in the pleural cavity.

In this erect view there is a horizontal straight line due to fluid (hollow arrow) with air above it. Whenever there is a horizontal line like this, it indicates that there is fluid with air above it, either in the pleural space or in a lung cavity.

# PULMONARY COLLAPSE (ATELECTASIS)

Collapse may involve the whole lung, a lobe of the lung (lobar collapse), or it may be patchy with only small segments of the lung being affected (segmental or subsegmental collapse).

*Collapse can be due to:*

(a) Blockage of a bronchus by intrinsic or extrinsic mass, foreign body, or aspiration.

(b) Compression of the lung by air or fluid in the pleural cavity.

*Collapse is diagnosed by:*

(a) Increased density and crowding of the pulmonary vessels.

(b) Displacement (upwards or downwards) of a hilum or fissure (the right hilum is normally situated at a lower level than the left).

(c) Shift of the trachea, mediastinum, or interlobar fissure towards the collapsed part of the lung.

(d) The remainder of the lung may become overexpanded and hypertranslucent.

The lower lobes are most likely to collapse: the increased density of a collapsed lung is not always visible in both projections, unlike pneumonia or fluid.

## Collapsed Right Upper Lobe

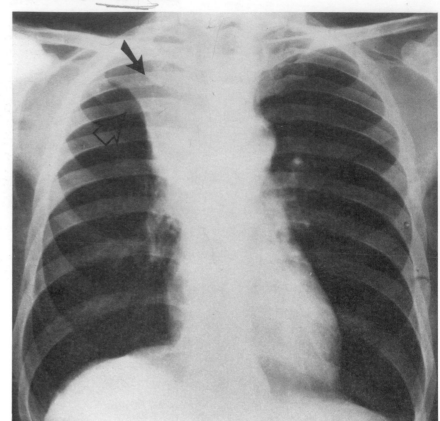

*PA view*

Uniform density of collapsed and shrunken right upper lobe (black arrow).

Right horizontal interlobar fissure rotated upwards towards the mediastinum (hollow arrow).

The right hilum is level with the left and is therefore elevated.

*Lateral view*

The collapsed lobe is not seen. This will help you to differentiate it from pneumonia: wherever there is consolidation it can be seen in both views, but collapse may be visible in only one.

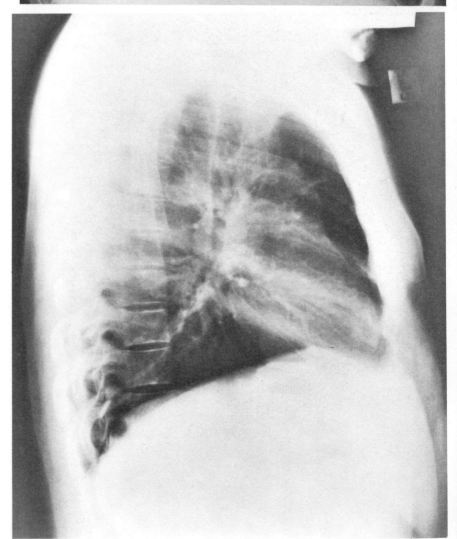

## Collapsed Right Middle Lobe

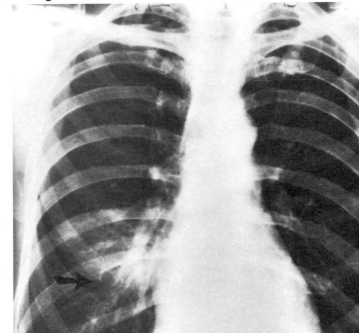

*PA view*

There is a density next to the heart in the right mid-zone, below the hilum. It is roughly triangular in shape. The lungs are otherwise clear.

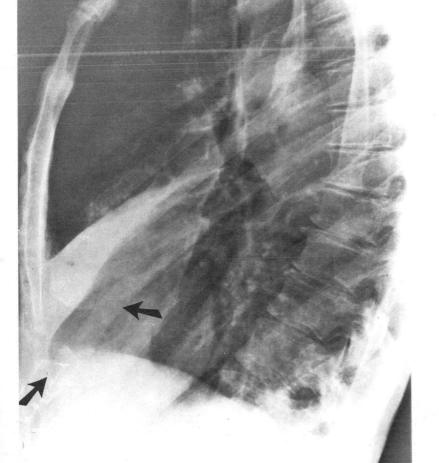

*Lateral view*

Middle lobe collapse is always more obvious in the lateral view, especially in children.

There is a triangular density anteriorly, indicating collapse of the middle lobe (black arrows).

## Collapsed Right Lower Lobe

*PA view*

Hypertranslucent right upper lobe due to compensatory increase in volume.

The right lower lobe has collapsed against the heart and mediastinum (arrows) obliterating the cardiophrenic angle. The line has a well-defined lateral boundary. The right hilum has "disappeared" because the pulmonary vessels have moved towards the heart as the lung collapsed.

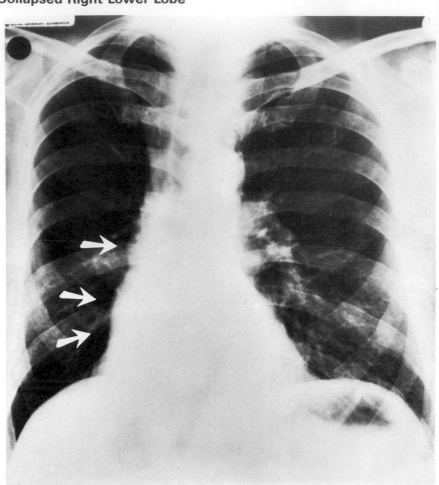

## Collapse of Both Right Middle and Lower Lobes

*PA view*

Hypertranslucent right upper lobe (hollow arrow).

As compared with collapse of the right lower lobe by itself, density on this film is larger and the outline is much less sharp.

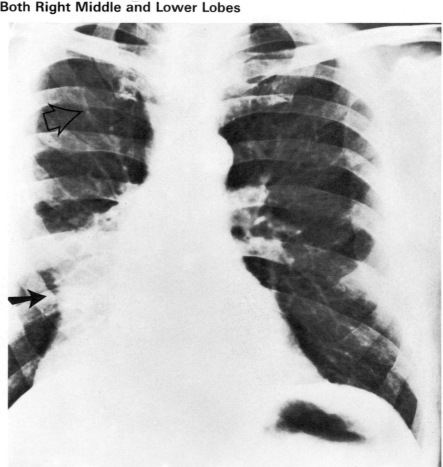

## Collapsed Left Lower Lobe

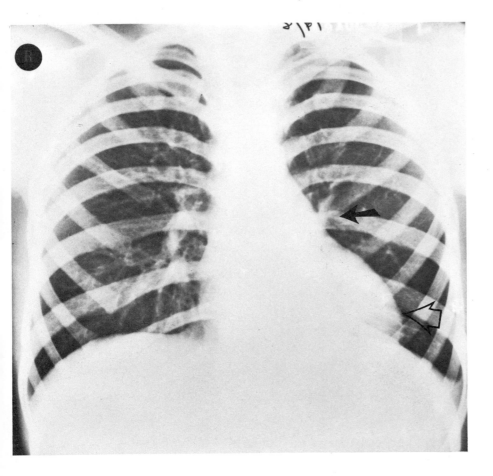

*PA view*

Slight cardiac and mediastinal shift to the left.

The left hilum is depressed below the level of the right hilum (black arrow).

There are decreased vascular markings in an overexpanded part of the left lung (hollow arrow). The collapsed left lower lobe is not seen in this inadequately penetrated view (see better exposure below).

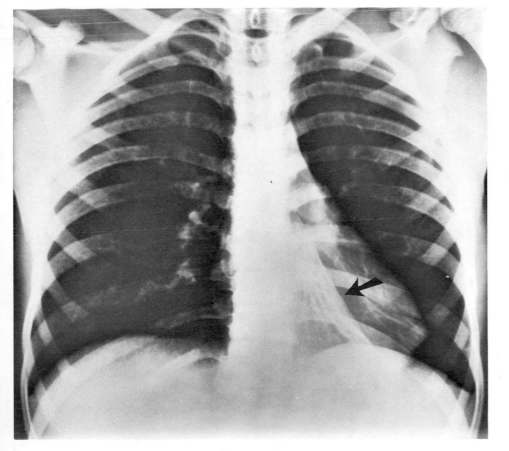

*PA view (same patient)*

To obtain this type of film, use basic PA chest technique but double the value of the mA·s.

Well-defined triangular density behind the heart is the collapsed left lower lobe (arrow). It is usually difficult to see a collapsed lower lobe in the lateral view.

## Collapsed Left Upper Lobe

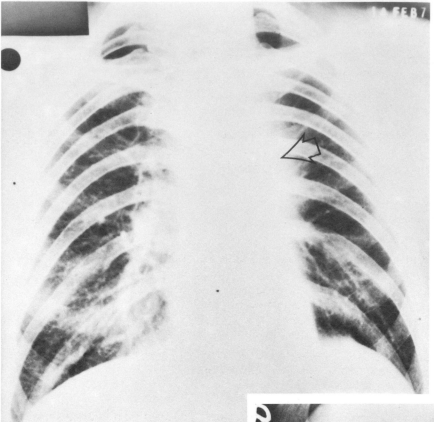

*PA view*

The left upper lobe has collapsed against the mediastinum (hollow arrow).

The mediastinum is slightly displaced to the left: on the left side the lung vessels are more spread out than on the right, owing to the compensatory overinflation of the remainder of the left lung.

*Lateral view*

The collapsed left upper lobe is difficult to identify because it has collapsed against the mediastinum. The posterior edge is evident (arrow).

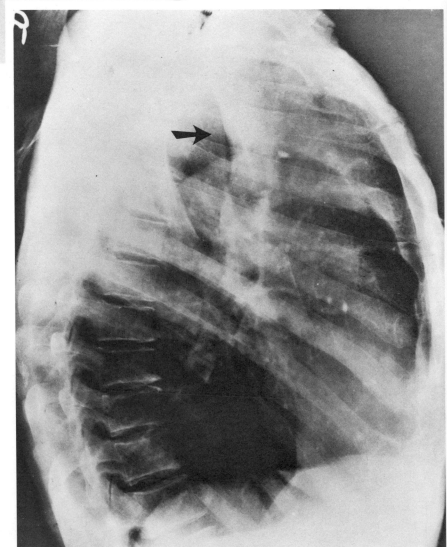

# DENSITIES IN THE LUNGS

First make sure that the density really is in the patient and not external. Examine the patient, remove clothing and exclude other external artefacts such as hair and skin lesions.

## Acute

If the patient presents with cough and fever of recent origin, consider:
(a) Pneumonia (see pages 52-55).
(b) Tuberculosis and other granulomatous disease (see pages 58-62).
(c) Lung abscess (see pages 56-57).

## Chronic

The patient presents with cough and often complains of excess sputum: there is usually slight fever and there may occasionally be clubbing of the fingers.
Consider:

(a) Pulmonary tuberculosis (see pages 58-62).
(b) Lung abscess (see pages 56-57).
(c) Tumour (primary or secondary, see pages 70–71), inhaled foreign body in children, or any other cause of bronchial obstruction causing collapse (pages 40, 45, 49-50).
(d) Bronchiectasis.

Always check the patient's occupational exposure and exposure to possible allergens (sick pets, etc.).

Diffuse and patchy densities in the lung have many different causes and the exact nature can be difficult to determine radiologically. Lung oedema due to cardiac or renal causes (or for any other reason) can result in patchy densities but in these patients fever is less likely. The chest film appearance should always be correlated with the clinical condition of the patient. If the film is difficult to interpret, send it, together with the clinical history, for specialist interpretation.

---

A DENSITY IN THE LUNG MAY BE DUE TO CONSOLIDATION, COLLAPSE, FLUID, OR TUMOUR. THE POSITION AND SHAPE OF THE DENSITY HELP YOU TO DECIDE WHICH IS THE CAUSE IN EACH PATIENT.

## Pneumonia (Inflammatory Consolidation)

When the air in the alveoli is replaced by any inflammatory exudate, that portion of the lung appears white on an X-ray. This may involve part or all of a lobe (lobar pneumonia), or may be patchy, involving the alveoli diffusely (bronchopneumonia). If the patch of pneumonia does not disappear in a month, further investigation is needed to exclude tuberculosis or underlying tumours.

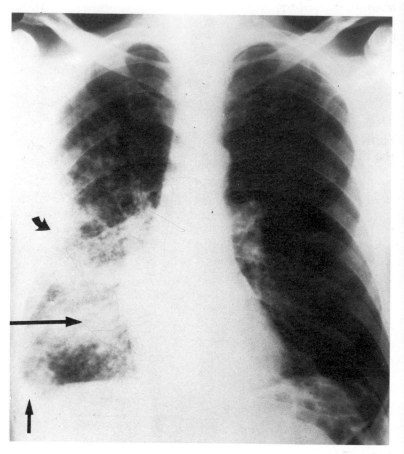

*Lobar pneumonia*

Peripheral consolidation.

Middle lobe consolidation

Small pleural effusion filling the costophrenic angle.

*Bronchopneumonia*

Severe bilateral bronchopneumonia: there are diffuse patchy densities throughout both lungs. Bronchopneumonia may be bilateral, as in this case, but may be restricted to only one part of a lung. It may be due to many different infections, including tuberculosis.

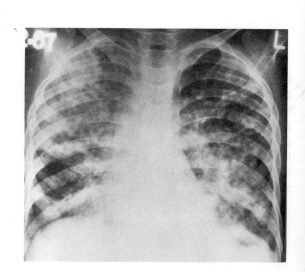

## Pneumonic Consolidation—Right Upper Lobe

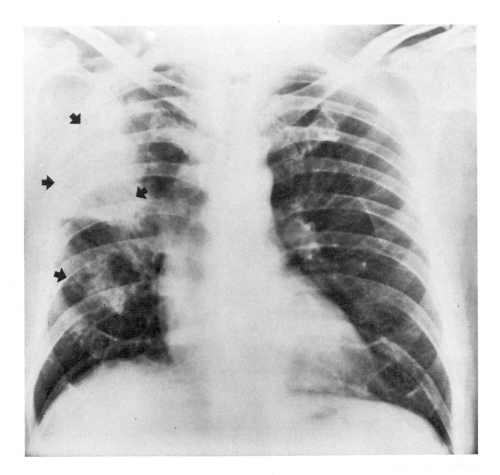

*PA view*

Dense opacity with in-definite outlines and accentuation of the air in some of the bronchi (air bronchogram).

Further consolidation in the right middle lobe.

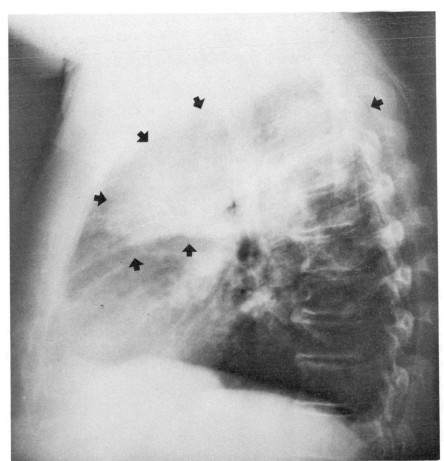

*Lateral view*

Dense consolidation in the upper lobe.

Note the sharp boundary of the interlobar fissures between the middle and upper lobe. The sharp line separating the right upper lobe and the right middle lobe is the horizontal fissure.

## Staphylococcal Pneumonia

Staphylococcal pneumonia has two different radiological patterns.

In some acutely ill patients there will be a severe destructive bronchopneumonia, often bilateral (see below). In others there are multiple small areas of consolidation, which are roughly round, hazy in outline and scattered through the lungs (this pattern may occur in staphylococcal pyaemia associated with osteomyelitis, for example). Pseudo-abscesses (tension cysts) then develop around the edge of the consolidation: they are not true lung abscesses because there is no breakdown of lung tissue, but are the result of bronchial obstruction. The walls are usually thin. There are often fluid levels within the cysts, but there may be very few clinical symptoms.

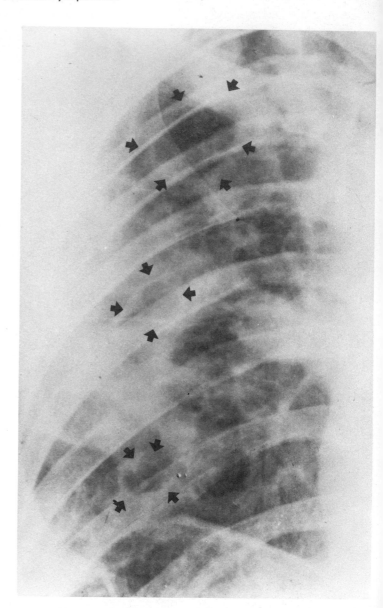

*Severe destructive bronchopneumonia*

This is usually due to a staphylococcal infection, but can also be caused by tuberculosis or chickenpox (varicella). Only ADULTS get chickenpox pneumonia, and they will be very ill.

This patient has numerous patches of consolidation with several thin-walled cavities, and has a high fever.

Such cavities strongly suggest a staphylococcal infection, which was the etiology in this case.

## Development of a Staphylococcal Pneumatocele

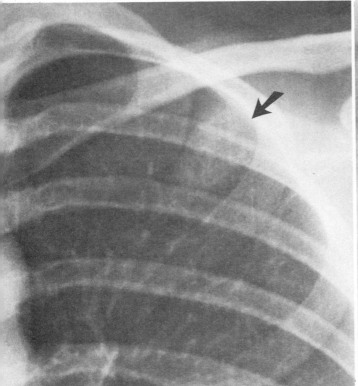

(a) Segmental solid area of consolidation.

(b) Pseudo-cavity develops from bronchial obstruction.

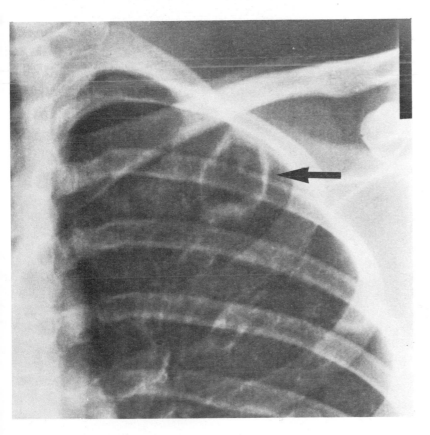

(c) Cystic cavity with thin walls in left upper lobe.

Nevertheless, these appearances CAN be seen also in tuberculosis or other granulomatous diseases. Bacteriological confirmation is essential before treatment is started.

## Bacterial Pulmonary (Lung) Abscess

Pyogenic lung abscesses may follow any severe infection, or inhalation of vomit or other irritating fluid or material, e.g., food. They may occur in any part of the lungs.

*PA and lateral views of a large abscess in the right lower lobe*

There is a fluid level: either the abscess communicates with a bronchus OR the abscess is caused by a gas-forming organism.

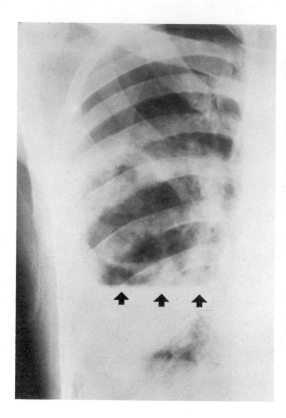
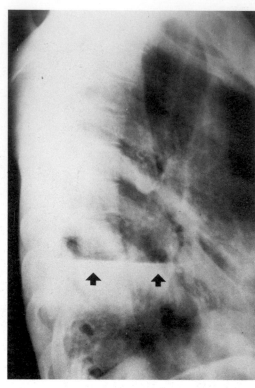

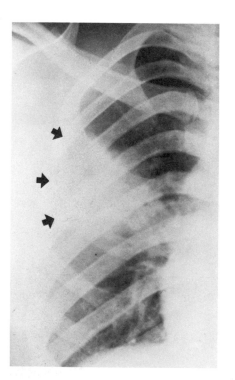

*Abscess following pneumonia*

Lobar pneumonia may become necrotic centrally and a lung abscess may follow.
In this patient the acute pneumonia in the posterior segment of the right upper lobe developed a central translucent area, most easily seen in the lateral view, which reveals the abscess with a thick irregular wall showing an air–fluid level.

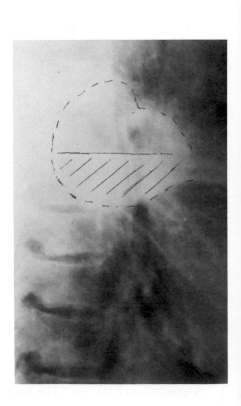

If an abscess fails to respond to appropriate treatment (some abscesses may take weeks to clear with antibiotics, but should show signs of improvement during the treatment), the possibility of an underlying tumour must be considered.

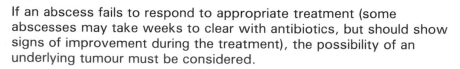

## Amoebic Lung Abscess

Pyogenic lung abscesses usually follow pneumonia or aspiration (e.g., vomit or foreign body). Amoebic abscesses are nearly all in the lower lobes, although they can occur anywhere in the lungs, especially in children. When either side of the diaphragm is raised, there is basal lung infection or lung abscess, and the liver is enlarged and sometimes tender clinically, then amoebiasis should be suspected.

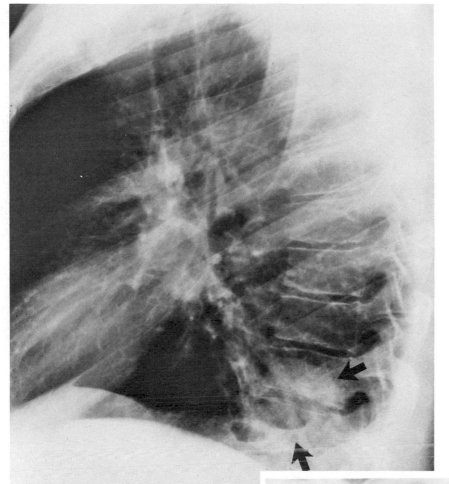

*Lateral view*

There is an inflammatory mass adjacent to the right diaphragm with central breakdown (arrow). All abscesses may appear solid at times, because of the contained pus. An air–fluid level within the abscess indicates that there is communication with the bronchus.

*PA view*

Abscess cavity with a fluid level (same patient).

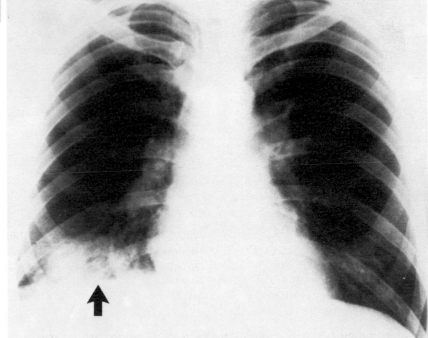

THE CAUSAL ORGANISM OF A LUNG ABSCESS CANNOT BE DETERMINED BY RADIOLOGICAL APPEARANCES (SEE ALSO TUBERCULOUS CAVITIES, pages 58–59).

## Acute Tuberculous Cavitation

Thin-walled cavity with surrounding tuberculous exudation.

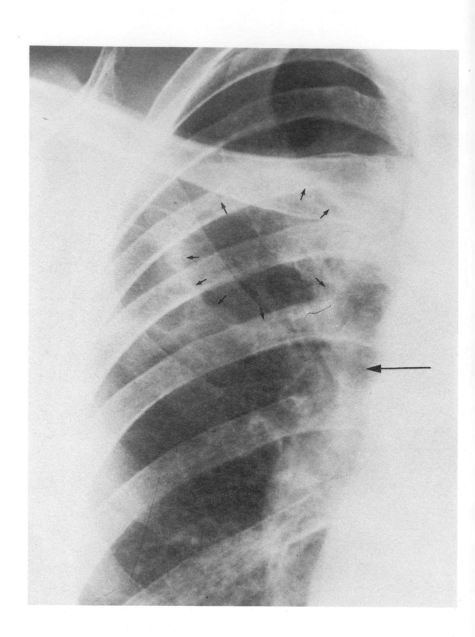

Increase in lung markings
extending to hilum, indicating
lymphadenitis (arrow).

Cavities may form quite early in tuberculous infection of the lung and may persist. When the cavity becomes chronic, the walls thicken and the cavity usually shrinks, followed by fibrosis. However, cavities vary even when the patient is on treatment, and they are not a good indication of his progress. Clinical indications are more important.

Multiple cavities in adults are most commonly due to tuberculosis. In childhood they can be tuberculous OR staphylococcal in origin. In areas where other diseases exist (e.g., paragonimiasis, melioidosis, histoplasmosis, coccidioidomycosis, blastomycosis) similar cavitation may occur which is not tuberculous: bacteriological confirmation must be obtained. Differentiation on radiological evidence alone is unreliable.

## Pulmonary Tuberculosis with Cavity Formation

Tuberculous infection spreads through the lungs and there may be multiple cavities, most commonly (but not only) in the upper lobes.

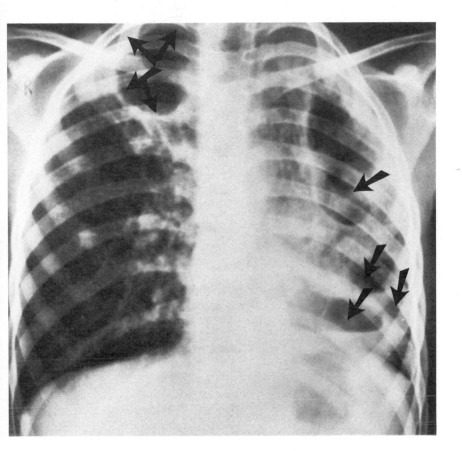

*Multiple cavities*

There are multiple cavities in the left lung and a large cavity in the right upper lobe. The volume of the left half of the chest is less than that of the right, an indication that the disease is chronic.

The progress of the disease cannot be assessed from a single film and even serial films may be misleading. Clinical judgement is most important, and repeated bacteriological examination is essential to assess activity or quiescence of the disease. Mechanical factors influence the size and fluid content of cavities, which fluctuate throughout the course of the disease.

If there is a density within the cavity, see also page 72.

CAVITATION AND FIBROSIS DO NOT ALWAYS MEAN **ACTIVE** TUBERCULOSIS.

## Massive Cavity Formation in Tuberculosis

Adult chronic pulmonary tuberculosis is a chronic granulomatous disease which causes extensive cavities and fibrosis (see note on page 51).

Almost all of the right upper lobe has been destroyed to form a large cavity.

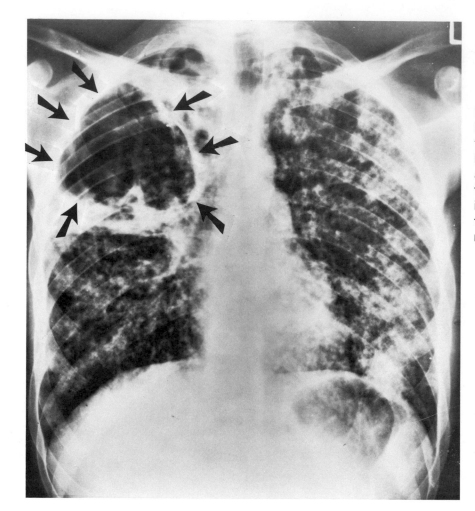

Patchy granulomatous changes throughout the left lung. These are probably the result of spill infection from the cavity in the right upper lobe.

Radiologically it is difficult to distinguish the various granulomatous diseases. Knowledge of local prevalence is all important in determining the most likely cause. Examination of the sputum is essential.

## Hydropneumothorax with Tuberculosis

A pneumothorax with or without effusion may develop in pulmonary tuberculosis or other granulomatous diseases. Persistence of a pneumothorax indicates the need for referral for further investigation to exclude bronchopulmonary fistula.

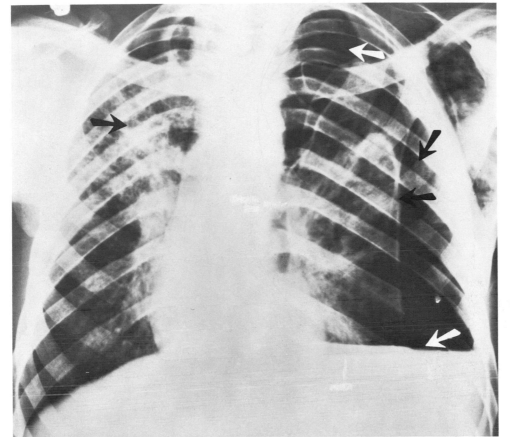

Tuberculosis causing patchy densities.

Heart displaced to right side by tension pneumothorax on left.

Pneumothorax.

Partly collapsed left lung.

Fluid at base of pleura.

Pneumothorax is an unusual complication of tuberculosis in adults, but is a little more common in children. It is always a serious complication that requires treatment.

## Miliary Tuberculosis

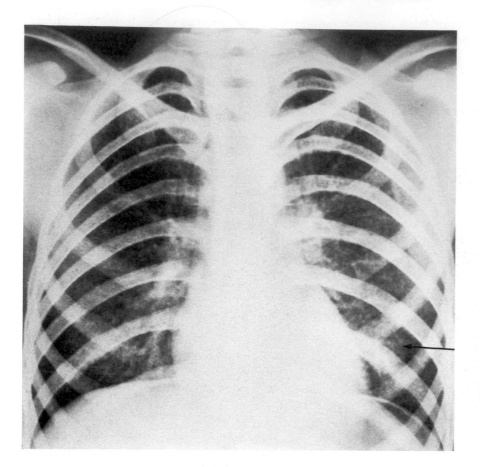

In tuberculosis and other granulomatous diseases, the miliary
nodules are seen throughout the
lungs.

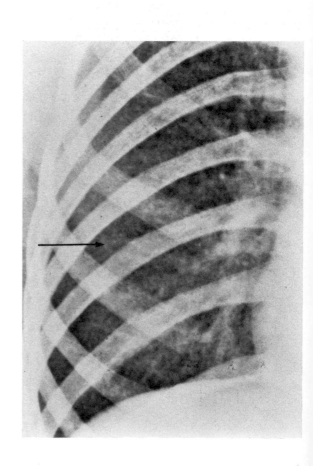

A detailed view of the right lung base showing the
small fluffy "soft" shadows.

There are very many causes of miliary nodules.

## Multiple Calcified Nodules

Calcification in nodules in the lungs must be recognized by the increased density of the nodules, which are often almost white. The edges of the margins are often clear cut.

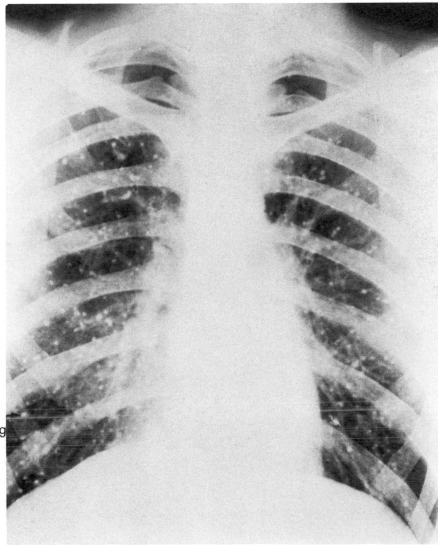

There is a diffuse spread of nodules throughout lung fields.

Small rounded calcified nodules with no surrounding pulmonary reaction.

Multiple small calcified nodules in the lung fields may be due to histoplasmosis and, more rarely, other granulomatous diseases, including chickenpox pneumonia (varicella). Miliary tuberculosis seldom calcifies like this.

Solitary or scanty calcified nodules are usually due to healed tuberculosis or other granulomas.

# ENLARGED LYMPH NODES

Lymph nodes are situated where the main bronchi divide and along each side of the trachea. When normal they are never visible on an X-ray. When they enlarge, the rounded outline of the nodes can be seen in the mediastinum and hila, as shown below. The lateral view may also be helpful.

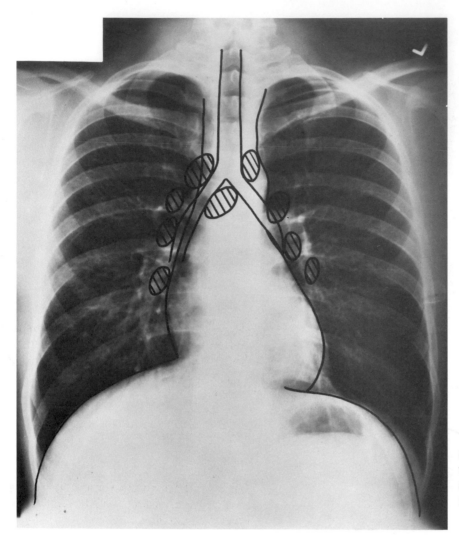

This radiograph and the drawing below show the typical appearance of hilar and mediastinal lymph nodes.

If there are large lymph nodes when the tuberculin skin test is negative, suspect sarcoidosis or lymphoma, especially when there is no response to antituberculous treatment.

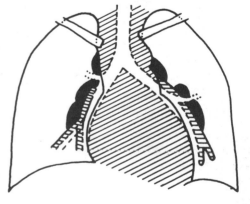

When there is calcification in hila or mediastinal lymph nodes, the cause may be:

(1) Tuberculosis or other granulomas, especially sarcoidosis.
(2) Silicosis or other types of pneumonoconiosis.

But the relevance of this finding must be assessed clinically and by laboratory tests.

## Tuberculosis

There are usually enlarged lymph nodes during the primary infection with tuberculosis. These nodes may be in the hilum or mediastinum. The tuberculous lung focus may not always be visible. The lymph nodes may be unilateral or bilateral. In children the lymphadenopathy may be best seen in the lateral view.

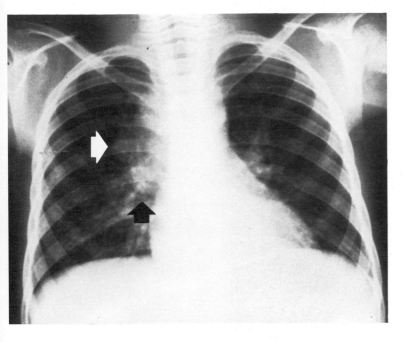

*Child*

Enlarged right hilar nodes (arrows). The primary infection in the lung is not visible.

Tuberculosis should always be suspected when a patient has pneumonia and enlarged lymph nodes can be seen radiographically.

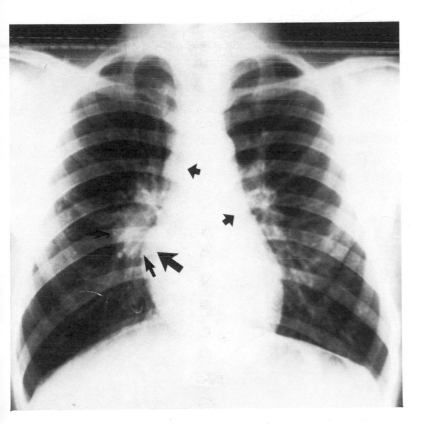

*Adult*

Bilateral hilar enlargement due to tuberculosis (the sputum may be negative for tubercle bacilli).

Hilar lymphadenopathy may be due to other causes, e.g., lymphoma or sarcoidosis. If there is no response to standard antituberculosis treatment, the patient should be referred for further investigation.

## ROUNDED PULMONARY DENSITIES

Round densities may be a chance finding on X-ray film, or be discovered because of cough or other chest symptoms.

### Round and clearly defined densities

(1) Primary or secondary malignancy (pages 70–71). Rarely, benign mass.
(2) Loculated effusion (page 43).
(3) Hydatid cyst (pages 68–69).
(4) Granulomatous disease, e.g., tuberculosis.
(5) Lung abscess (pages 56–57).
(6) If near the spine, a neurofibroma is possible.

### Calcification in the wall of the density

(7) A dermoid cyst (usually mediastinal) (page 67).
(8) In the upper chest; may be the thyroid.
(9) Close to the apices of the chest or mediastinum; may be an aneurysm of the great vessels or of the aorta (page 79).
(10) Calcification can occur in the pericardium following infection (tuberculosis or rheumatic fever).

Hydatid and pericardial cysts do not usually calcify in the lung.

### Calcification in the nodule (not just in the periphery)

(1) It may be a granuloma (tuberculosis, etc.). Assess activity clinically.
(2) It may be a benign tumour. It is not usually malignant.

)N IN ANY NODULE WITHIN THE CHEST INDICATES THAT IT IS VERY UNLIKELY TO BE MALIGNANT.

## Dermoid and Other Calcified Cysts

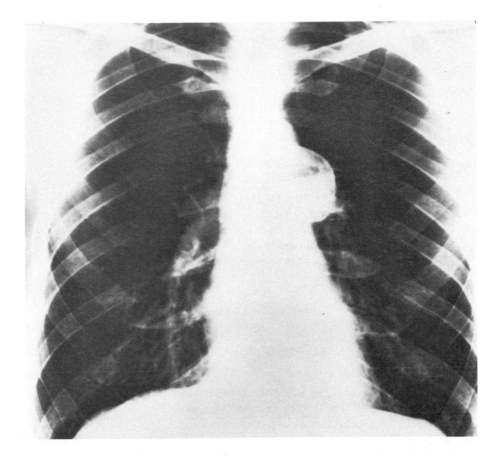

*PA view*

A calcified ring shadow projects from the left side of the mediastinum. A lateral view is therefore essential to localize it.

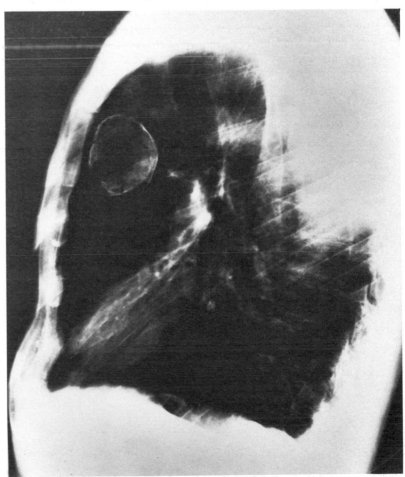

*Lateral view (same patient)*

The calcified ring shadow is in the anterior mediastinum; this is a common site for dermoid tumours.

## Hydatid Cysts

Hydatid cysts may be of any size and may be single or multiple. They are usually spherical and smooth, without lung reaction around them. They can be solid, or hollow with a fluid level.

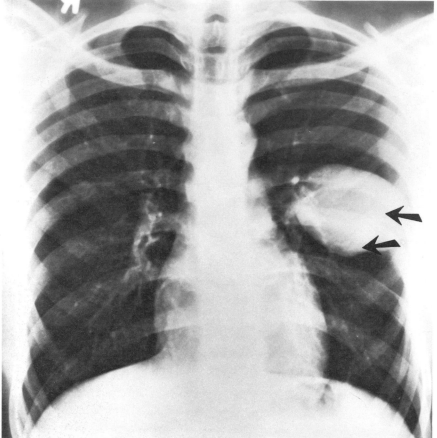

*A solid unruptured cyst*

Note the smooth outline and the lack of surrounding pulmonary reaction. These cysts may appear slightly lobulated.

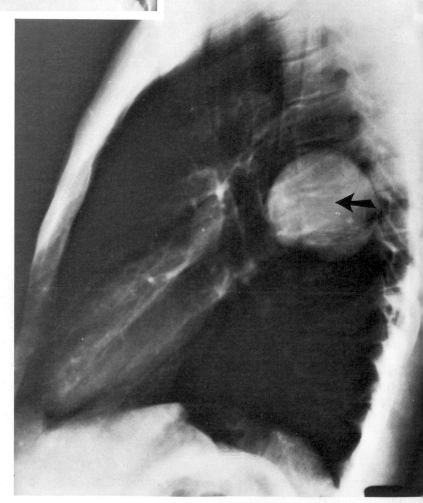

*Lateral view (same patient)*

The smooth outline and homogeneous density indicate that this is a cyst full of fluid. There is no pleural or pulmonary reaction.

(An interlobar effusion (page 43) may slightly resemble a hydatid cyst, but there is never a fluid level when fluid is in a fissure. Look carefully for the fissure to make the differential diagnosis. Fluid usually changes within a few days; hydatid cysts do not alter until after a few months.)

If the fluid from a hydatid cyst spills into the pleural cavity, the patient may have a very serious "shock" reaction.

## Hydatid Cysts (continued)

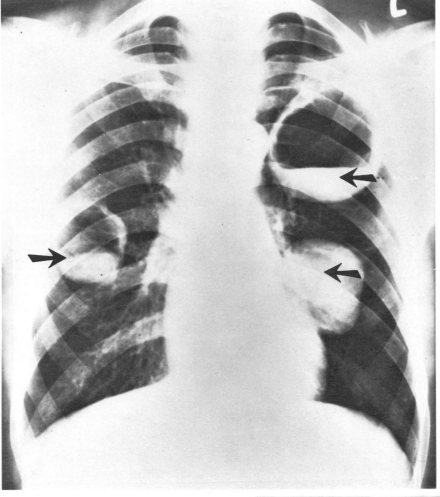

*PA view*

Three cysts in the same patient. The lower cyst on the left appears solid; the other two cysts are communicating with bronchi and some of the contents have been coughed up, leaving fluid with a fluid level in each.

The lower cyst has not ruptured and has clearly defined outlines.

*Lateral view (same patient)*

A ruptured cyst with a fluid level. This is in the left upper lobe (see PA view).

A ruptured cyst with a daughter cyst within it. This is in the right lower lobe.

The solid cyst which has not ruptured (white arrow) lies anteriorly on the left side.

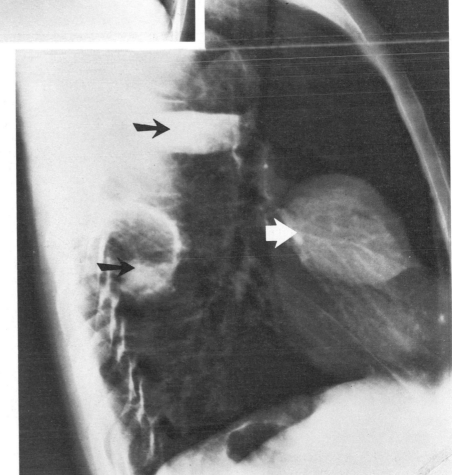

Occasionally when the hydatid cyst ruptures into a bronchus it subsequently becomes infected causing foul sputum and a fever.

## Primary Lung Cancer

Cancer in the lung may appear as a solitary round shadow or may cause collapse of a lobe of the lung because the tumour blocks a bronchus. Early cancers can be very small and irregular in outline, but they sometimes become smooth as they grow larger.

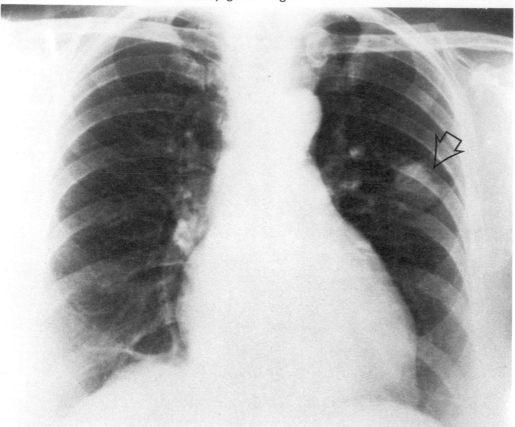

*Solitary nodule*

Single, round, uniform density, with clear margins. There is no calcification.

Lung cancers may show a small dimple (notch) somewhere on the margin.

In this patient there is little or no surrounding lung reaction.

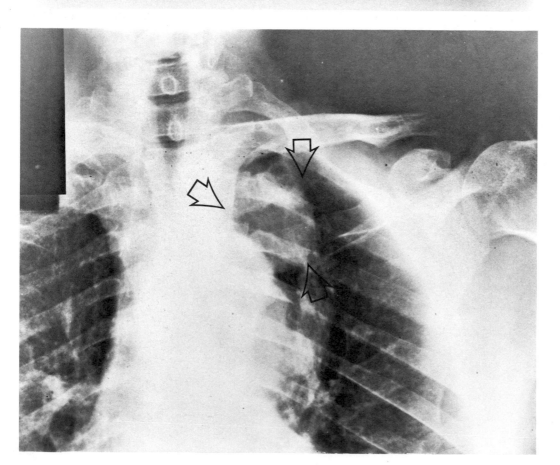

*Carcinoma in the apex of the lung*

There is a round homogeneous mass (hollow arrows) but no lung reaction. This may be in the lung tissue or adherent to the mediastinum. When tumours are high in the apex of the lung they may cause pain because they involve the pleura or the rib.

## Secondary (Metastatic) Lung Cancer

The radiological features of secondary lung cancer give NO indication of the site of the primary growth.

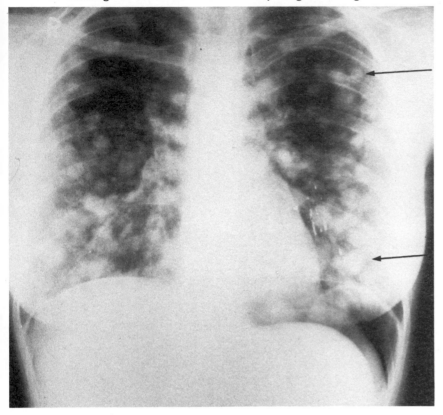

*Multiple metastases*

Opacities of varying size with clearly defined edges, except where the masses overlap each other. Look for destructive lesions in bone, indicating other metastatic deposits.

This type of metastasis may occasionally cavitate.

The hilar lymph nodes are usually normal.

Metastases may occasionally be single, but are more often multiple and of different sizes.

*Chorioepithelioma*

Occurs ONLY in women of childbearing age. The secondary deposits (shown below) may be smooth but can have ill-defined edges suggesting infection. In the early stages it can resemble miliary tuberculosis. The lymph nodes remain normal.

A similar appearance may be seen in many other conditions (see page 66).

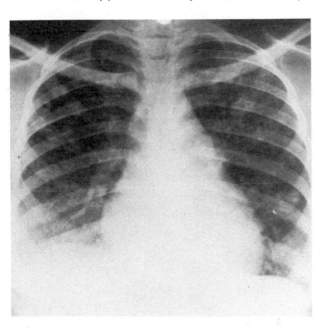

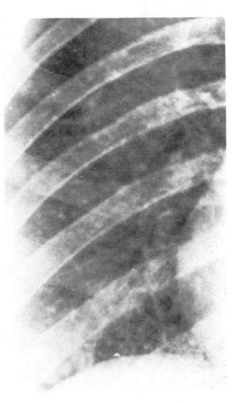

## Mycetoma (Fungus Ball)

Chronic cavities in the lungs can become infected by a fungus, such as *Aspergillus,* which then forms a rounded mass within the cavity. Such mycotic infections most frequently occur in chronic, fibrotic tuberculous cavities.

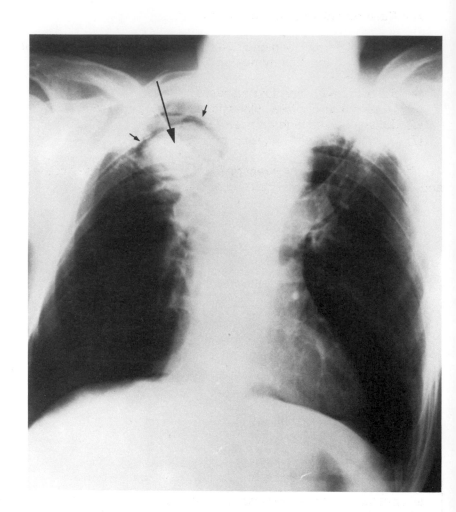

*PA view*

A dense mycetoma almost filling a large cavity at the apex of the right lung (long arrow).

The smaller arrows indicate air between the cavity wall and the fungus ball within it. If the patient is X-rayed in the decubitus position, these fungus balls usually change position.

# DIFFUSE INCREASE IN LUNG PATTERN (A "RETICULAR" PATTERN)

An increased reticular "network" pattern throughout both lungs has multiple etiologies. It is seldom possible to make an exact diagnosis from the X-ray film alone.

A diffuse reticular pattern can occur in:

(1) Early pulmonary oedema (may change in a short period of time).
(2) Carcinoma invading lymphatics.
(3) Sarcoidosis.
(4) Silicosis and other dust diseases.
(5) Tropical eosinophilia: filariasis and other parasites.
(6) Collagen disease (e.g., rheumatoid).
(7) Fibrosing alveolitis (in response to allergens).

There are more than 40 recognized diseases which may cause this reticular pattern throughout the lung and expert opinion may therefore be needed!

---

BE CAREFUL. A FILM TAKEN IN POOR INSPIRATION OR UNDEREXPOSED (TOO LIGHT) CAN SUGGEST AN INCREASED RETICULAR PATTERN (pages 32–33).

## Pneumoconiosis (Industrial Disease)

Inhalation of some dusts may result in pulmonary fibrosis. Silica is especially dangerous, causing silicosis.

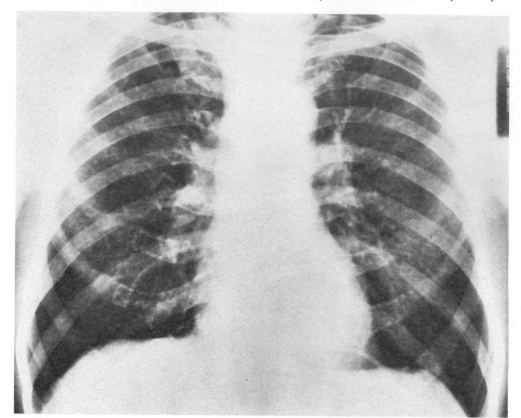

*Silicosis*

This starts as a fine reticular pattern and progresses to fine nodule formation, resembling miliary tuberculosis, but most marked in each lung below the clavicles. Eventually large nodules may occur (massive fibrosis), also in the upper zone. The hilar lymph nodes may enlarge and calcify (see facing page).

The early stages of silicosis cause a fine reticular pattern in the upper part of each lung. This can be mimicked by poor inspiration. Small nodules then appear in each lung (small arrows), followed by larger nodules (hollow arrow).

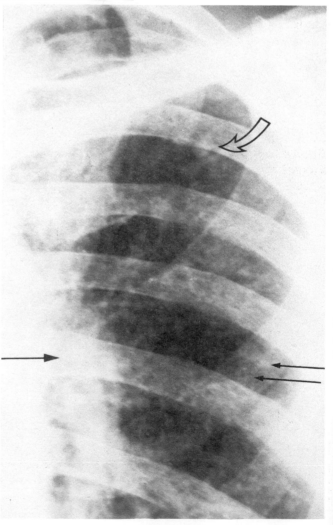

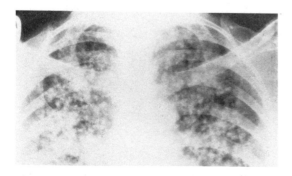

In some patients the nodules calcify: they are always most numerous under the clavicles, and always bilateral, but not necessarily exactly symmetrical.

### Pneumoconiosis *(continued)*

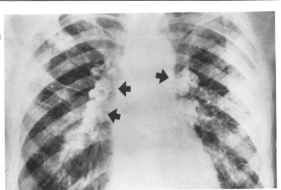

*Calcification of the hilar lymph nodes due to silicosis*

This pattern of eggshell calcification is only seen in silicosis or sarcoidosis. Tuberculosis and other granulomatous diseases calcify the nodes into solid densities, not the hollow, eggshell pattern seen here.

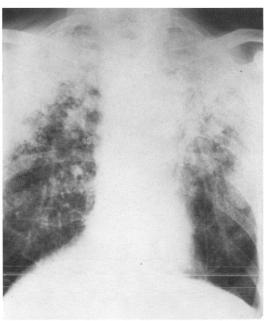

*Advanced silicosis*

This causes massive fibrosis—always bilateral but not always the same on each side. It is always more severe in the upper part of each lung, with elevation of the hila and overexpansion of the lower lobes (emphysema).

This can be differentiated from metastases because of the severe fibrosis and contraction, which is not seen when there are nodular metastases. Although some of the "masses" may resemble a primary carcinoma of the lung, the masses in silicosis are always multiple and bilateral.

Chronic but active tuberculosis is often associated with silicosis and the sputum must be examined numerous times to exclude this infection.

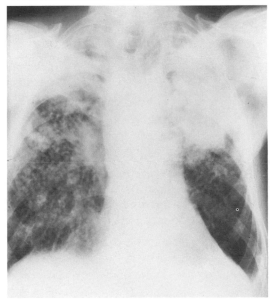

THESE RADIOLOGICAL FINDINGS ARE NOT SPECIFIC. IF THERE IS NO MINING OR INDUSTRIAL EXPOSURE, CONSIDER OTHER ALLERGENS—ASBESTOS OR SUGAR CANE, FOR EXAMPLE, AMONG MANY POSSIBLE SUBSTANCES—OR OTHER CONDITIONS, SUCH AS FARMERS' LUNG.

# THE HEART

## Normal Heart Borders

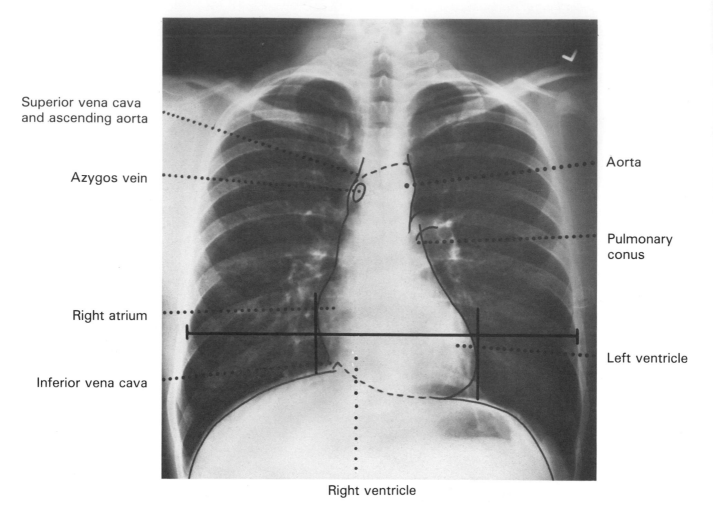

Superior vena cava and ascending aorta

Azygos vein

Right atrium

Inferior vena cava

Aorta

Pulmonary conus

Left ventricle

Right ventricle

If heart failure is diagnosed clinically, X-ray examination usually adds little further information.

*Heart size and shape*

The width (transverse diameter) of the normal adult heart in the PA projection is less than half the maximum width of the chest. But to assess this, the film must be taken in full inspiration with the patient in the erect position. This is an approximate indicator.

The heart may appear normal on X-ray even when there is good clinical evidence of valvular disease, arrhythmias, coronary thrombosis, coronary artery disease, or congenital heart disease. A normal chest X-ray does *not* exclude cardiac disease.

As the films on page 78 demonstrate, it can be very difficult to distinguish a cardiomyopathy from pericardial fluid. In most cases with pericardial effusion, the pulmonary vessels will be less visible than usual because of decreased cardiac output. A rapid increase in the size of the heart, or a rapid decrease after treatment, suggests that the large cardiac shadow is the result of a pericardial effusion.

Apart from this, the distinction must be made clinically.

*Enlarged heart*

The commonest causes are:

    ...ertensive heart disease.
    ...umatic and other valvular diseases.
    ...t cardiomyopathies.
    ...cardial effusions (collections of fluid).
    ...e cases of congenital heart disease in children and adults.

## Lateral View of Heart

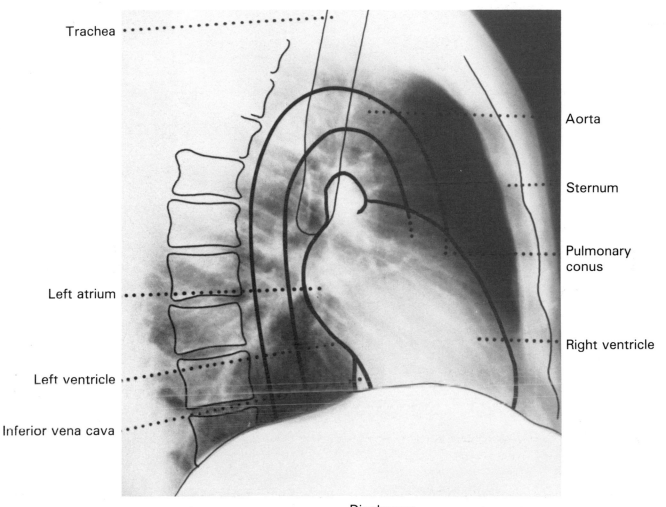

Trachea

Aorta

Sternum

Pulmonary
conus

Left atrium

Right ventricle

Left ventricle

Inferior vena cava

Diaphragm

A LATERAL PROJECTION IS NEEDED WHEN THE HEART IS ENLARGED ON THE PA FILM. ONLY BY LOOKING AT BOTH THE PA AND THE LATERAL FILMS CAN THE ENLARGED CARDIAC CHAMBERS BE CORRECTLY IDENTIFIED. THIS CAN SOME-TIMES BE DIFFICULT, PARTICULARLY IN CHILDREN. (FULL INSPIRATION AND A TRUE LATERAL PROJECTION ARE NEEDED.)

## Pericardial Effusion and Cardiomyopathy

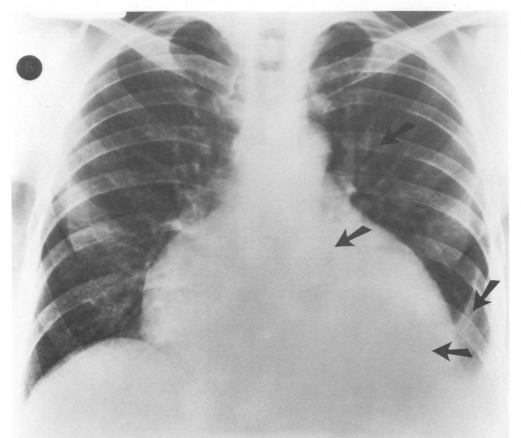

*Pericardial effusion*

Normal lung vessels.

Grossly enlarged globular cardiac outline.

Left pleural effusion.

Pericardial effusion.

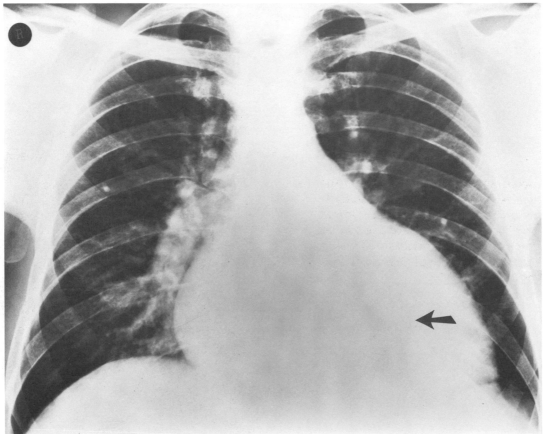

*Cardiomyopathy*

The pulmonary vessels are usually prominent.

Generalized cardiac enlargement.

These two conditions are shown together to emphasize how difficult it can be to tell them apart.

## Aortic Aneurysm

Aortic aneurysms can be very difficult to differentiate from a mediastinal mass, such as a carcinoma. Both PA and lateral projections are necessary, but even then will not always be conclusive.

Following trauma, a widened mediastinum may indicate damage to the aorta or great vessels. It needs referral for further investigation.

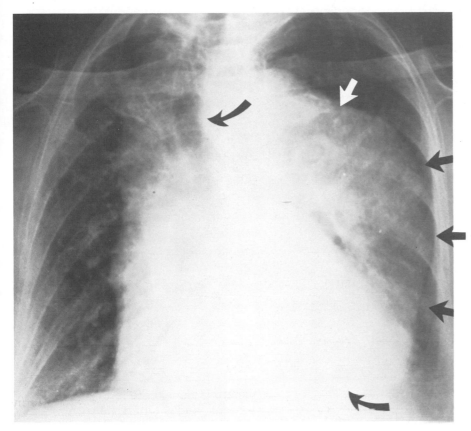

Displaced trachea (curved arrow).

Calcification in wall of aorta (white arrow).

Dense smooth shadow of dilated descending aorta (arrows).

Large heart.

*A very large aortic aneurysm (syphilis)*

*Another, smaller, aneurysm*

If you suspect an aortic aneurysm, try to identify the outline of the aorta: this will usually be smooth and well defined. (Many tumours are shaggy in outline and poorly defined.) Look for displacement of the trachea, almost always to the right, by an aneurysm. Try to identify any calcification in the wall of the aorta. A lateral view may help.

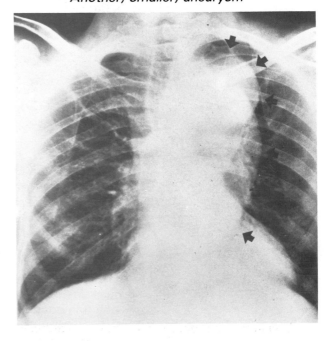

## Pulmonary Oedema

Oedema of the lungs associated with a large heart is usually due to cardiac failure. If the heart size is normal, the oedema may result from renal failure or fluid overload (excess intravenous fluid). Characteristically, pulmonary oedema alters rapidly with treatment or may change with the patient's position. There are often pleural effusions. Pulmonary oedema may be of pulmonary origin—e.g., mountain sickness, drowning, smoke inhalation, or inhalation of toxic gases.

Pulmonary oedema can change into adult respiratory distress syndrome (shock lung) and it can be very difficult to separate the two conditions radiologically. When oedema fails to respond to the proper treatment with diuretics, etc., adult respiratory distress syndrome (ARDS) should be considered.

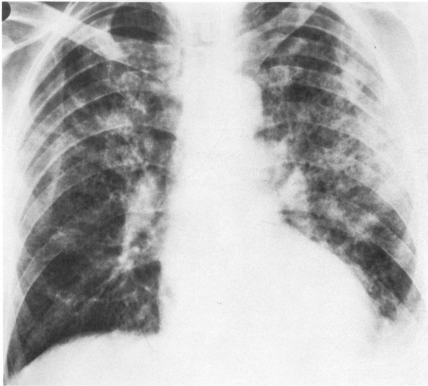

Patchy oedema in both lungs. Bilateral, but unevenly distributed: the densities are different shapes (not lobar) and ill defined.

There is fluid in the left costophrenic angle. Often there are bilateral effusions.

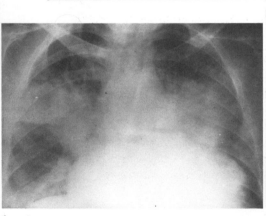

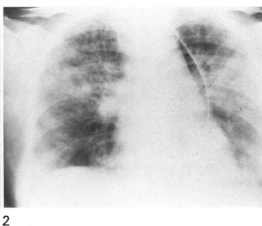

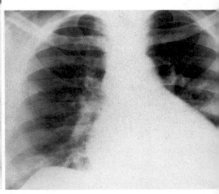

1                                2                                3

(1) Severe pulmonary oedema due to excess intravenous fluid. Can also occur as a result of renal failure, heart failure, drugs, and, rarely, malaria.

(2) The same patient the next day, following diuretics and fluid restriction.

(3) The same patient one week later. Rapid change and quick response to treatment is characteristic of oedema. Infection does not alter in this way.

These films were all taken with the patient sitting in bed.

## CHESTS OF INFANTS AND YOUNG CHILDREN

The chest films of infants and young children differ in many ways from those of adults. Some of the differences are due to the difficulties of obtaining a good inspiratory film, as well as to anatomical differences between the age groups.

In children:

(1) The bony thorax is broader and the ribs are more transverse.
(2) The diaphragms are higher and the superior mediastinum appears wider.
(3) The heart has a more globular character: heart size cannot be accurately judged in relation to the size of the chest.
(4) The width of the superior mediastinum may be exaggerated by a persistent thymus, usually projecting on to the right lung (particularly in infants who are crying) but occasionally seen on the left (see pages 82–83).

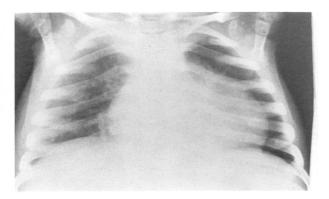

*Normal child's chest X-ray (erect)*

Although it appears very large, the heart is quite NORMAL.

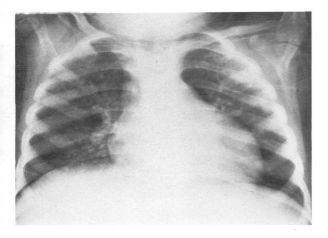

*Another normal child's chest X-ray (erect)*

The heart size and shape are normal for a child of this size. There are normal lung markings and normal hilar shadows. The upper mediastinal width is also normal. The depth of inspiration is not so great as it should be in an adult erect chest.

(The circle over the left upper chest is due to a button—not a cavity in the lung! Clothing and hair often cause confusing shadows.)

## Technical Fault—Poor Inspiration

A child's chest X-rayed during *expiration*. The right lower lobe is so compressed that it resembles an area of pneumonia. The heart and mediastinum are very wide and the lungs are so hazy that they look like cardiac failure or pulmonary oedema.

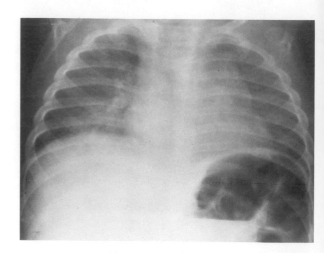

The same child re-X-rayed a few minutes later in full *inspiration*. The pneumonia is "cleared"! There is no longer any suggestion of pulmonary oedema and the heart size and shape are normal. The same radiographic technique was used, but the film looks "darker" because there is much more air in the lungs (air appears black on an X-ray).

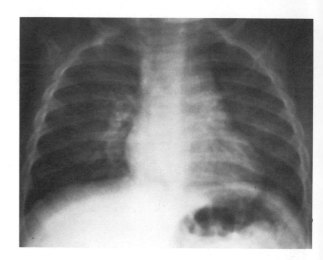

## Supine

A supine chest X-ray with the child's arms alongside the head.

The heart is enlarged and an unusual shape because it has spread out in the supine position and has curved over the thoracic spine. The upper-lobe pulmonary vessels are distended in this position (also in adults).

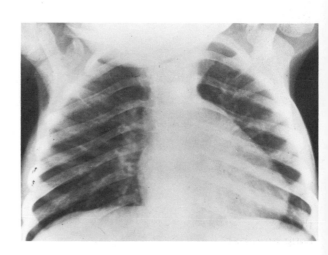

## Thymus

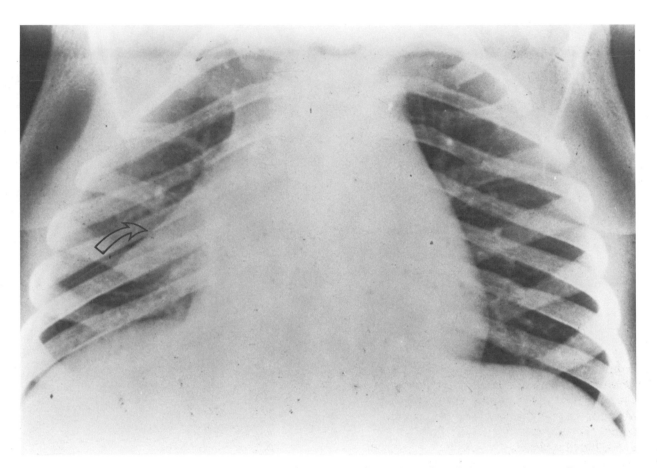

Triangular sail-like shadow of the thymus arising from the right side of the superior mediastinum.

*Inadvertent oblique position*

*PA view*

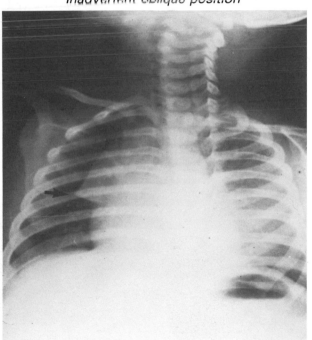

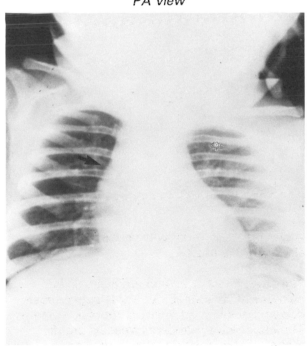

Same patient, same day.

Oblique film shows the sail-like shadow of the thymus projecting from the mediastinum and lying anteriorly.

Straight right border of superior mediastinum is the only indication of an enlarged thymus.

# SKELETAL X-RAYS

# SKELETAL X-RAYS*

## GENERAL PRINCIPLES

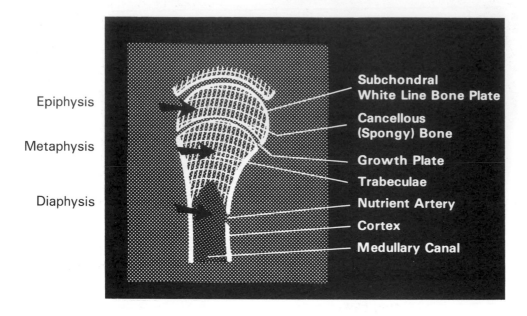

Epiphysis

Metaphysis

Diaphysis

Subchondral
White Line Bone Plate

Cancellous
(Spongy) Bone

Growth Plate

Trabeculae

Nutrient Artery

Cortex

Medullary Canal

**Glossary**

*Sclerosis.* The bone is dense, white.

*Trabeculae.* The woven pattern in a bone.

*Scalloped.* Wavy.

*Endosteal.* The inside of the cortical bone.

*Medulla.* The space filled with bone marrow.

To detect fractures and dislocations, one X-ray may not be enough:

(a) Obtain two views as nearly as possible at right angles for ALL suspected fractures and dislocations, except in the pelvis where oblique projections may help. Sometimes more views may be needed—e.g., the wrist—but look at the routine views first. (See the BRS *Manual of radiographic technique.* In the present book only one view has usually been provided, to save space.)

(b) Make sure that the films always show the joint ABOVE and BELOW any suspected fracture of the forearm or leg, unless it is clinically obvious that the injury is only in the most distal part of the limb. But even then, the nearest joint must be included.

(c) Remember that TENDON or VASCULAR damage cannot be seen on routine X-rays.

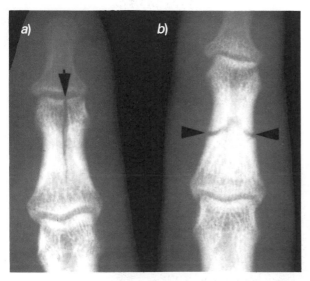

(a) *Vertical fissure, intra-articular fracture.*

(b) *Transverse fracture.*

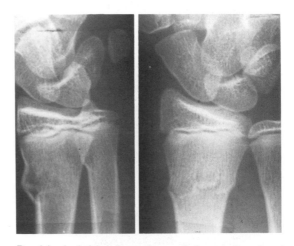

*Buckle (crinkle) fractures of the radius (and ulna).* A childhood injury.

---

* Section on skull, see pages 125–143; section on spine, see pages 145–155.

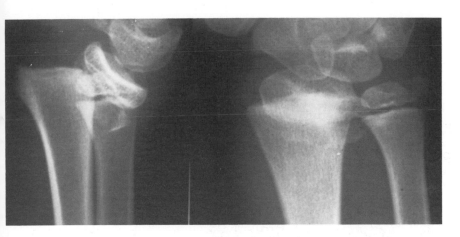

Displayed epiphyseal fracture.

Fractures of the shaft of bones can usually be easily seen when there is obvious displacement or a break in the thick cortex. In children, the cortex may buckle. A displaced epiphysis is usually easy to see.

However, with cancellous bone it may not be easy to recognize the fracture, unless.it is seen in profile (on edge). More than two views may be necessary—e.g., four views for a suspected scaphoid fracture (wrist)—but when any fracture is suspected, but not seen on the X-ray, re-examine the patient after 10 days if symptoms still persist. In the first week or two, a fracture line often becomes more obvious. After that the fracture unites, the line will disappear, and the bone reforms.

## Non-Union

It is important to recognize when a fracture has failed to unite, because surgery may be necessary. The fracture line persists, instead of disappearing. The broken ends of the bone become more white (sclerotic) and there is often thick new bone around the fracture, but this does not join together properly. There may be movement clinically.

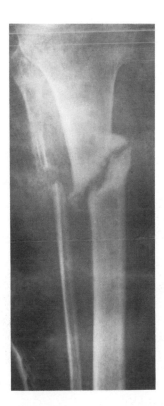

Both these fractures are "un united" and will not now unite simply by immobilization.

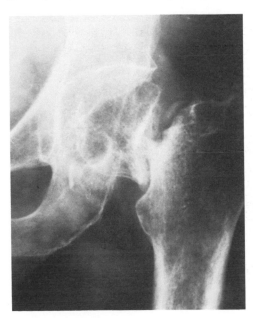

This tibial fracture may be separated by interposed soft tissue or as the result of therapeutic traction for too long.

## Multiple Injuries

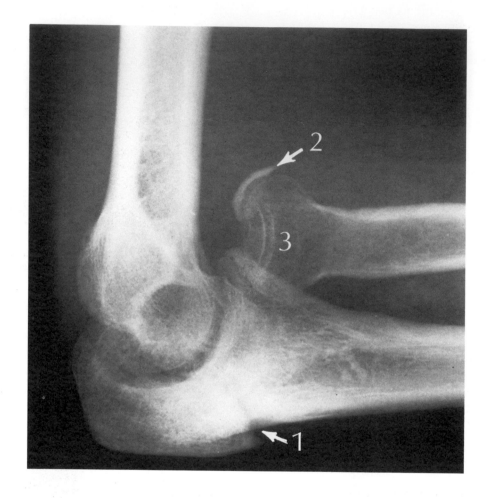

There are 3 injuries visible on this film:

(1) fracture through the olecranon;
(2) fracture of the radial head;
(3) dislocation (luxation) of the head of the radius.

When looking at an X-ray film, remember that because you have seen one obvious injury, you MUST NOT stop looking, as there may be further fractures or other abnormal findings.

In this instance, a further view at right angles (an AP projection) might have been helpful. In this type of injury, extension is limited by pain and protective spasm, so that only an imperfect AP could be obtained. But even such a view can be of diagnostic assistance. The radial head might be dislocated or there might be other linear fractures.

# TRAUMA

## Foreign Bodies

Only certain materials can be seen in the soft tissues:

*Usually visible*

Heavy metals such as lead, brass, and steel.
Coins.
Stone and rock.
Some injected drugs—iodine, bismuth, barium
and iron.

*Usually invisible*

Plastics.
Light metals, e.g., aluminium.
Glass, unless it is lead-containing.
Wood and thorns.

*Occasionally visible*

Glass with high lead content.
Overlying bandages and adhesive dressings.

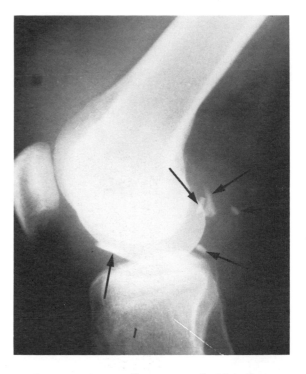

Patient fell through a skylight. The knee is swollen, a gas bubble from
the entry wound is in the tissues and many fragments of lead-containing
glass are in the joint (arrows). (Remember—air will appear black and
dense materials will appear white.)

Remember and recognize surgical clips and steel surgical sutures.
Remember also that an apparent foreign body may be on clothing: buttons, clips, items in pockets or on the skin. If you suspect this, check
the patient, clean the skin and remove clothing, and then re-X-ray if
necessary. Coils of hair or dirt in the hair may also make confusing
shadows.

*Technique*

Always have two views at right angles. If there is an entry wound,
fasten a marker on it, such as a needle or a straightened paper-clip;
If you suspect a foreign body in the eye, take frontal views using two
different cassettes. If an opacity is visible on both films, it is not an
artefact. Then take the lateral view of the face.

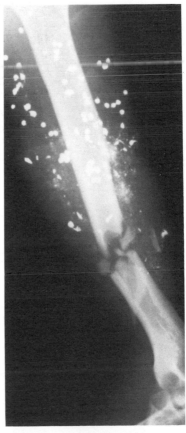

There are numerous lead gunshot pellets in the soft tissues. The
humerus is fractured and bone fragments also lie in the soft tissues.
The AP view would localize the pellets and show the angulation of the
fracture more completely.

## Hand—Terminal Phalanges*

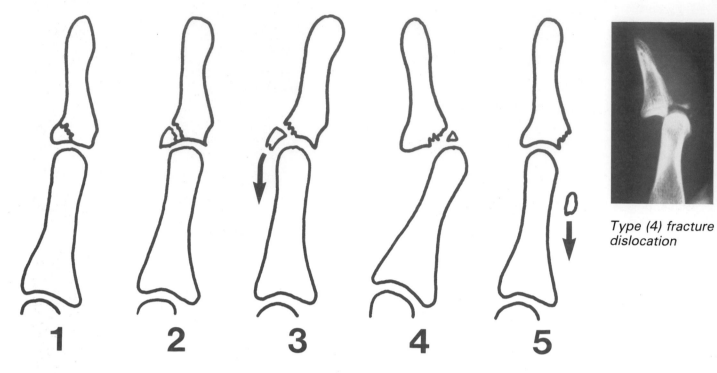

Type (4) fracture dislocation

(1, 2, 3) Lateral views of a finger with varying degrees of displacement of the posterior avulsion injuries by the extensor tendon. It is the loss of function of the tendon that is important, rather than the inconsequential-appearing fracture. The tendons cannot been on the film.

(4) Anterior detachment following a posterior dislocation.

(5) A fragment avulsed by the long flexor tendon. This injury requires surgical repair.

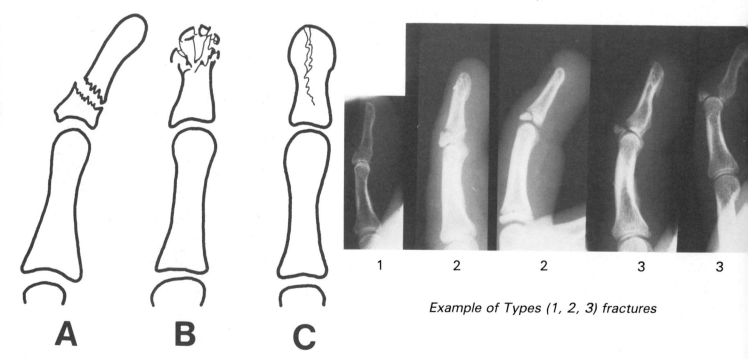

Example of Types (1, 2, 3) fractures

Varieties of fractures of the terminal tuft of the phalanx

---

* An X-ray taken after reduction should show almost complete restoration of normal anatomy, especially in adults. If it does not, refer for specialist opinion.

## Hand—Middle Phalanges

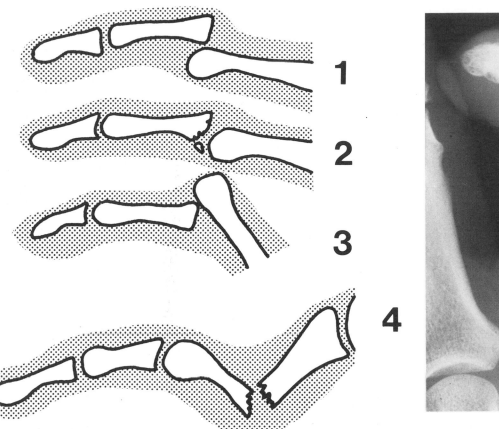

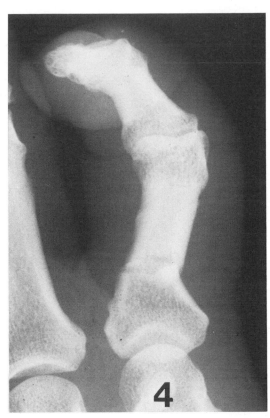

(1) Posterior dislocation of middle phalanx.
(2) Posterior dislocation with avulsion of volar cartilage plate and a bone fragment.
(3) Anterior dislocation.
(4) Angulated mid-shaft fracture.
(5) Oblique shaft fracture with rotation deformity.

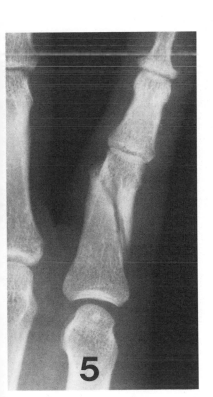

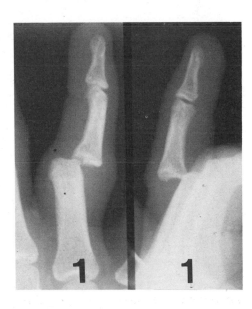

## Hand—Middle Phalanges *(continued)*

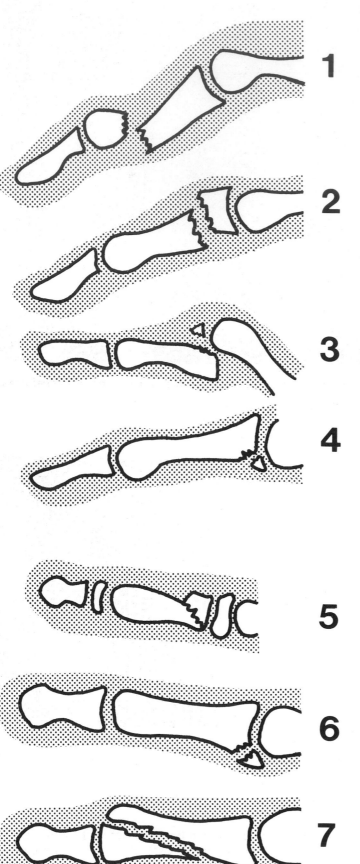

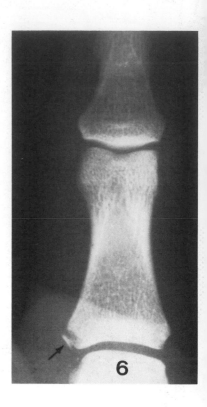

**1**

**2**

The diagrams indicate the typical fractures and dislocations that occur.

Remember: soft tissue, ligamentous, and tendon damage are invisible in radiographs.

**3**

**4**

**6**

**5**

**6**

**7**

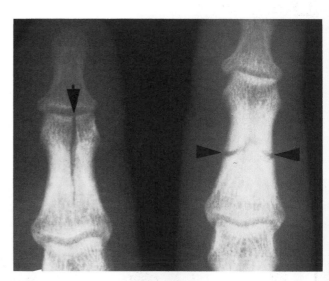

Vertical and transverse fractures of middle phalanges. The vertical fissure involves the joint.

## Metacarpal Fractures

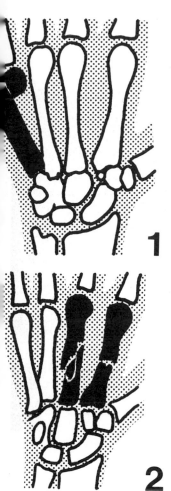

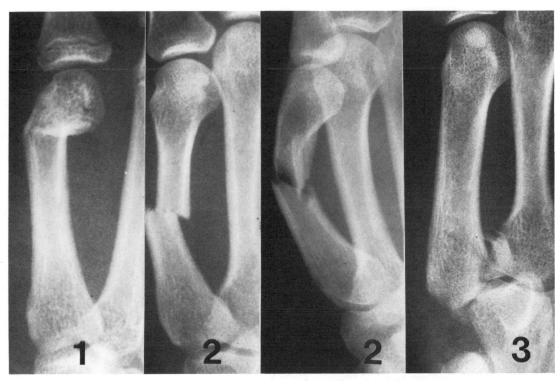

(1) The most common metacarpal fracture occurs in the distal metaphyseal area.

(2) The third metacarpal shows a spiral fracture of the shaft with rotation deformity. The second metacarpal transverse fracture usually becomes angulated.

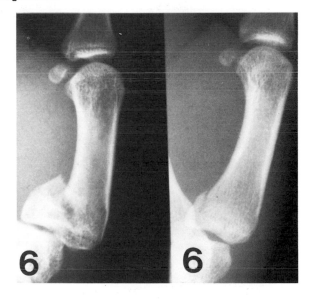

(3) A fracture at the base of the fifth metacarpal. Because of tendon pull, this is often unstable with proximal displacement.

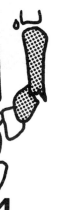
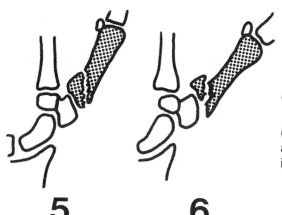
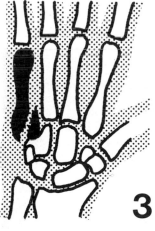

(4) Impacted angular fracture.

(5, 6) Oblique basal fractures (of first metacarpal) with and without proximal displacement. Accurate reduction is required.

## Thumb

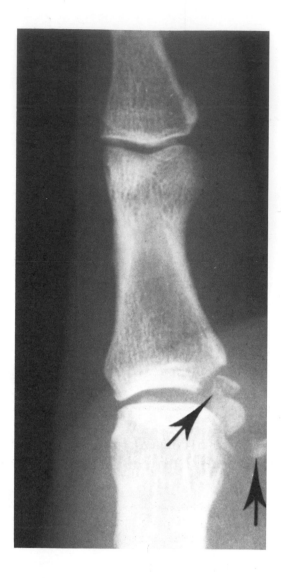

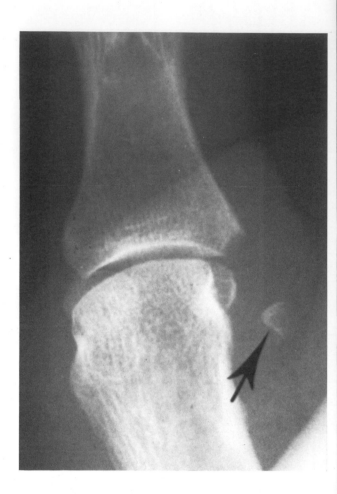

These two radiographs illustrate a *serious* injury of the thumb. If there is a greatly displaced fragment on the ulnar side of the base of the proximal phalanx of the thumb, this is a trapped avulsed fragment that requires open reduction, to make sure that the thumb is able to grip adequately in future.

SUCH CASES NEED OPEN SURGICAL REDUCTION

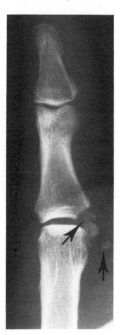

Since the enlargements (above) may confuse the reader,
one of the thumbs is shown natural size.

## Scaphoid Fractures

Scaphoid fractures may be difficult to detect. Multiple views are needed. You should be guided by clinical findings and immobilize. If symptoms persist, repeat examination two weeks later (without cast).

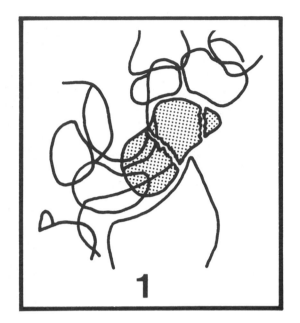

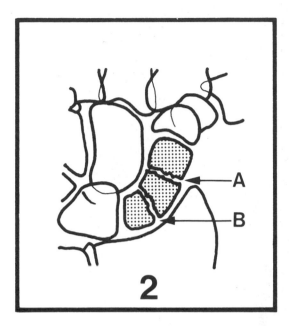

(1) This oblique view shows two fractures. One is the common fracture through the waist of the bone. The second is of the distal pole.

(2) Transverse fractures of the scaphoid are usually near the centre (A), but when proximal (B), they are more serious: the blood supply is poor and healing takes a long time.

(3) A fracture of the waist of the scaphoid.

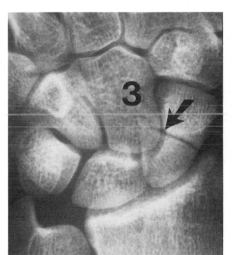

(4) Because of poor blood supply (note how dense the bone is where it has died proximally and the lucent repair zone distally), this will require prolonged treatment for healing and may need surgery.

## Carpal Dislocations

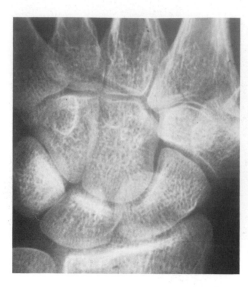

Radiographs showing normal PA wrist. The space between the radius and ulna and the first row of the carpus is a smooth curve. A similar curve exists between the proximal and second distal carpal bones. A smooth undulating line separates the distal carpal row and the metacarpal bones. If this is interrupted, suspect a dislocation.

It is important to recognize and reduce these lesions at an early stage.

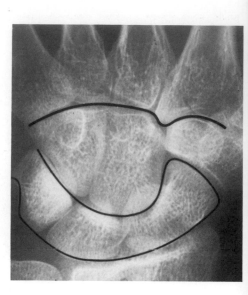

(1) Diagram of normal wrist PA and lateral.

In the following diagrams, the bones in abnormal position are shaded.

(2) Anterior dislocation of the lunate. Note the triangular shape in PA, and anterior displacement and rotation in lateral view.

(3) Perilunar dislocation. The lunate is a normal quadrilateral in PA view, but overlaps the capitate and is separated from the scaphoid. In lateral view, all carpal bones are displaced posteriorly.

(4) Trans-scaphoid perilunar dislocations resemble (3) above, except that there are fractures of the radial styloid and the waist of the scaphoid. In lateral view, the lunate is normally related to the radius and the capitate is displaced posteriorly.

## Carpal Dislocations *(continued)*

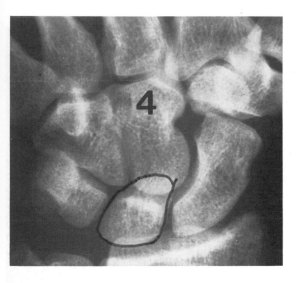

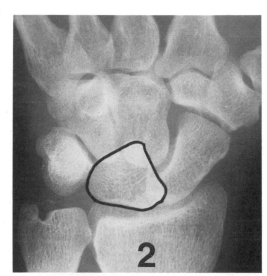

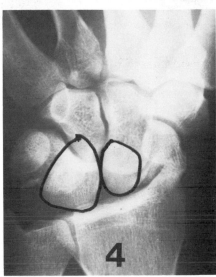

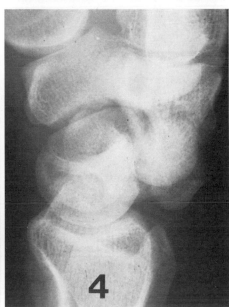

A normal wrist (1) with the lunate outlined. It has a curved triangular shape.

Compare the PA views of an anterior lunate dislocation (2) and a perilunar trans-scaphoid dislocation (4). (The numbers refer to diagrams on the facing page.)

*Lateral views*

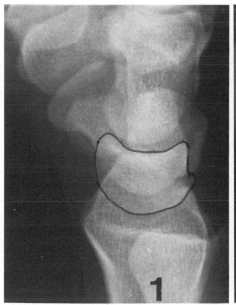

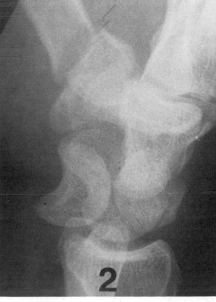

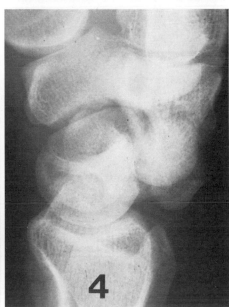

In the normal lateral view the lunate is again outlined. Its moon shape sits in the curve of the radius with the capitate fitting in the distal concavity (1). In an anterior lunate dislocation, the lunate is rotated 90 degrees (2). In a perilunate trans-scaphoid dislocation, the lunate maintains its radial articulation and the capitate is displaced posteriorly (4).

# Forearm

In all forearm injuries, always include on the film the ELBOW and WRIST JOINTS, as proximal or distal radio-ulnar dislocations will otherwise be missed.

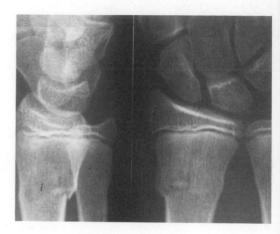

Buckle fractures of the radius and ulna

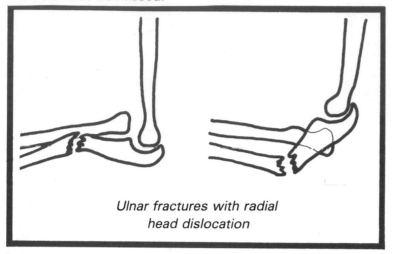

Ulnar fractures with radial head dislocation

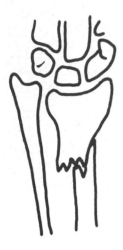

Distal fracture of radius
If there is no ulnar fracture, ensure that the distal or proximal radio-ulnar joint is not dislocated.
In such a proximal radial injury, views of the elbow should also be obtained.

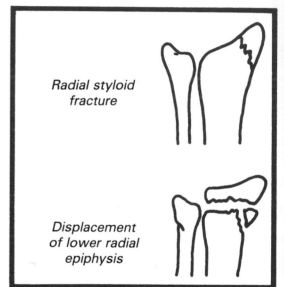

Radial styloid fracture

Displacement of lower radial epiphysis

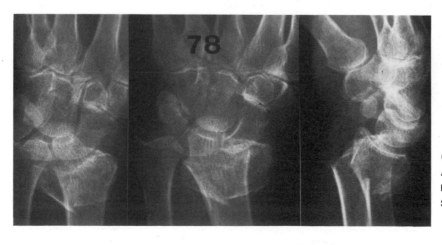

Comminuted Colles' fracture
A Colles' fracture of the distal radius with typical dorsal tilt and supination displacement.

**Elbow**

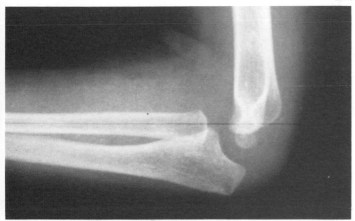

A line drawn parallel to the shaft of the radius should meet the midpoint of the capitellum. This radius is dislocated, as the intersection of the line with the humerus is too high.

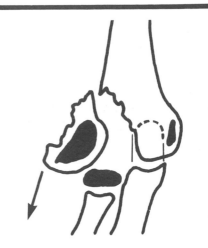

Lateral epicondyle displaced and rotated by pull of extensor muscles (arrow) in a child

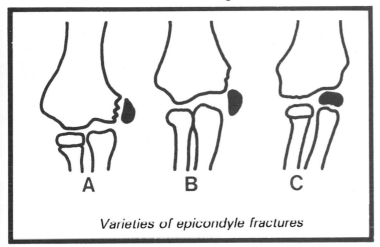

*Varieties of epicondyle fractures*

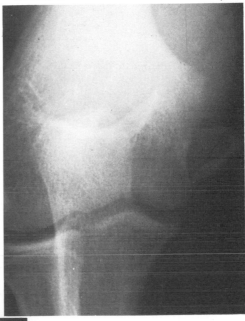

*Medial epicondyle fracture with some displacement*

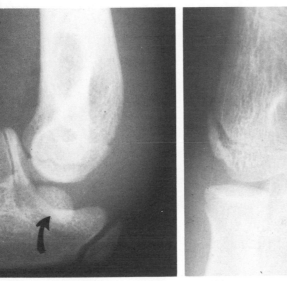

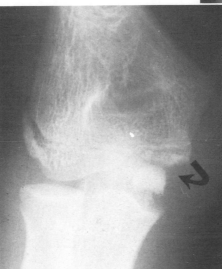

*AP and lateral views*

Fracture of medial epicondyle which is displaced intra-articularly (arrows point to trapped condyle).

IF THERE IS ANY DOUBT ABOUT ANY INJURY AROUND THE ELBOW OF A CHILD, X-RAY THE NORMAL (OPPOSITE) ELBOW FOR COMPARISON—SEE ALSO NEXT PAGE.

## Elbow *(continued)*

The approximate appearance of the elbow joint at different ages. This is to emphasize the need for a control comparison view of the normal elbow when in doubt after looking at the film of the injured elbow. (Numbers indicate age in years.)

Ages in years

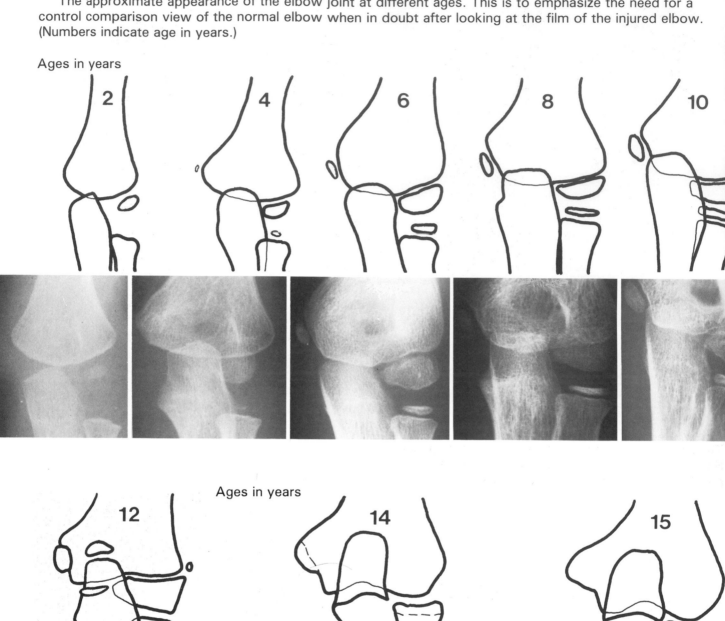

Ages in years

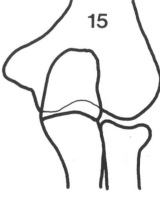

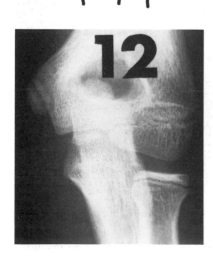

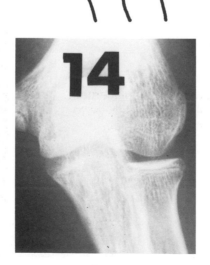

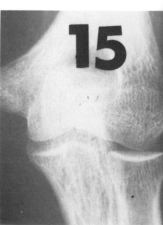

## Injuries of the Humerus

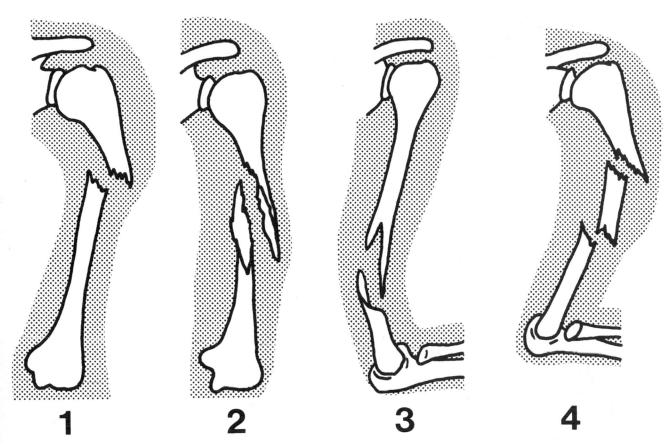

**1**      **2**      **3**      **4**

*(1)–(4) Various fractures of the shaft of the humerus.*
The rotational deformity can be severe with spiral fractures.
Some of these fractures cause vascular or neurological
problems. Check distal pulse and sensation.

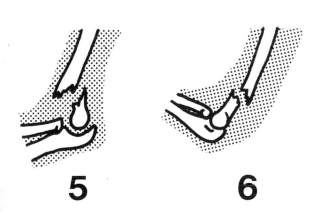

**5**      **6**

*(5, 6) Supracondylar fractures*
These fractures can have anterior or posterior displacement.
Vascular injury, due either to direct trauma to vessels or to
later swelling, makes these injuries potentially serious.

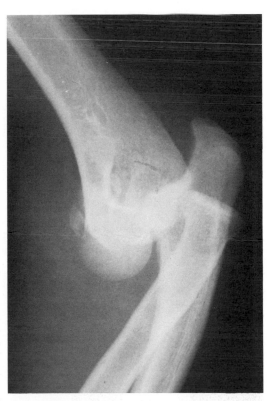

*Posterior dislocation (luxation) of elbow*
There is a detached fracture of the coronoid process of the
ulna. Remember possible vascular and neurological compli-
cations.

## Clavicle and Acromio–Clavicular Joint

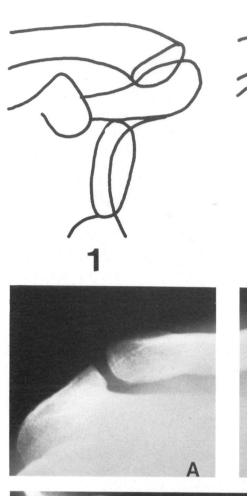

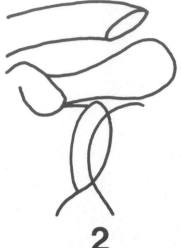

**1**

**2**

When the acromio–clavicular joint is injured, the major damage is usually to the ligament. X-ray the shoulders to exclude fractures and then repeat the X-ray with the patient holding weights in each hand. Compare the two sides. The width of the injured joint will increase if there is damage.

*(1) Normal acromio–clavicular joint*

*(2) Early dislocation. The joint space is widened*

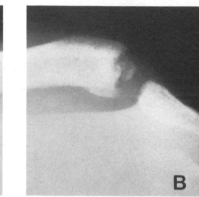

**A**

**B**

*(A) Normal acromio–clavicular joint*

*(B) Acromio–clavicular dislocation with fracture of the lateral part of the clavicle*

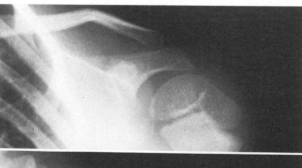

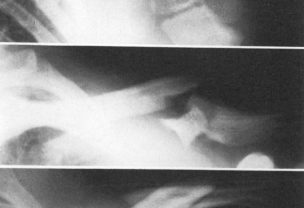

*Three examples of fractures of clavicle*

The upper is a greenstick, the middle has a separate central fragment and the lower is the most frequent midshaft type.

ONLY X-RAY THE CLAVICLE WHEN THE CLINICAL DIAGNOSIS OF A FRACTURE IS UNCERTAIN.

# Shoulder

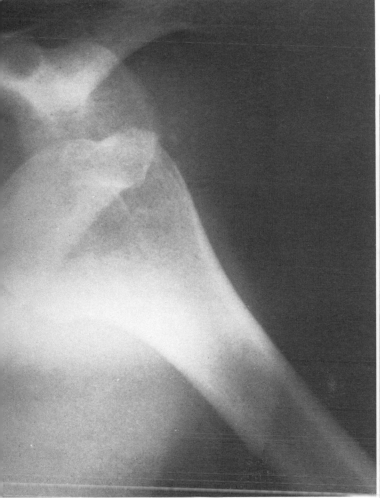

Anterior shoulder dislocation

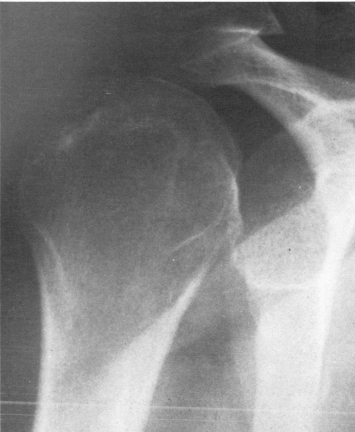

*Posterior shoulder dislocation*

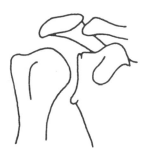

*Normal shoulder*

*Posterior
shoulder dislocation*

Look for any of these signs
of posterior dislocation.

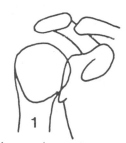

1

*Internal rotation*

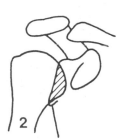

2

*Medial overlap*

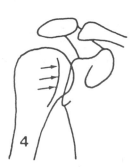

3

*Separation over 6 mm*

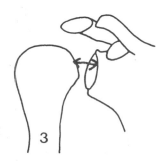

4

*Trough (depression)*

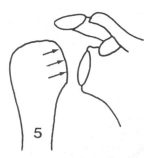

5

*Flattening*

**Shoulder** *(continued)*

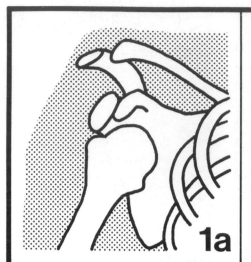
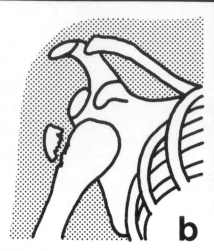

*(1a) Anterior dislocation of the shoulder*

*(1b) Anterior fracture–dislocation of the shoulder*
The greater tuberosity is detached.

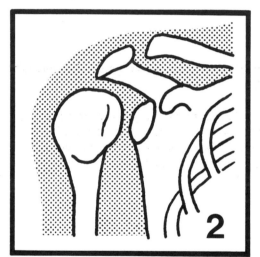

*(2) Posterior dislocation of the shoulder*

This dislocation can be easily missed. Note the internal rotation of the humerus. The patient cannot externally rotate the humerus.

Shoulder injuries need good clinical and radiological correlation.

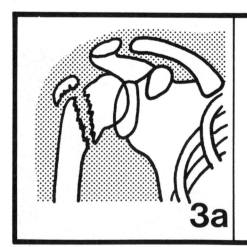
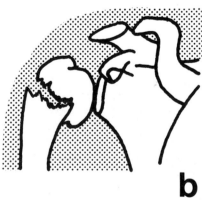
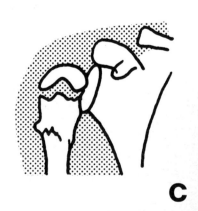

*(3a) Complex fractures of the humeral neck*
*(3b) Impacted fracture of the surgical neck of the humerus*
*(3c) Greenstick fracture of the upper humeral shaft in a child*
(The separate fragment is the normal epiphysis.)

**Shoulder** *(continued)*

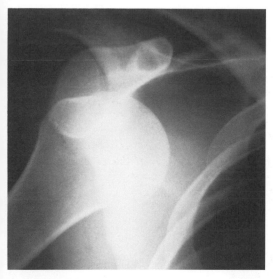

*(1a)* *Anterior dislocation*

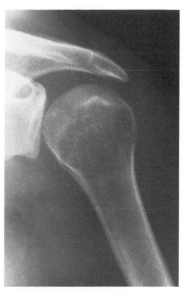

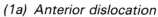

*(2)* *Posterior dislocations*

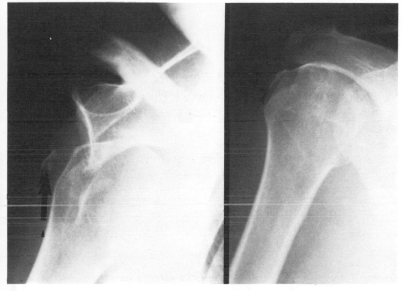

*(1b)* *Anterior dislocation*

Numbers refer to drawings on the opposite page.

With dislocations, fragments of bone can be avulsed. Reduction of the dislocation often results in approximation of the detached fragment.

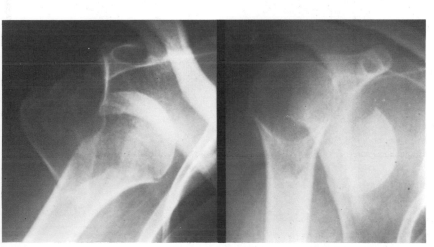

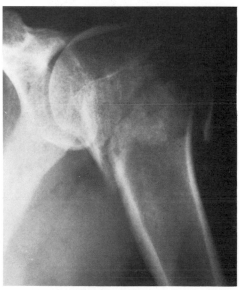

*(3a)* *Complicated fracture–dislocation*

## Pelvis

Most pelvic fractures are easy to see, but remember that they are almost always multiple. The pelvis is a bony ring interrupted at the sacro-iliac joints and the pubic symphysis. Trauma to the ring almost always causes two or more fractures. If you can only see one bony injury, look carefully at the joints and ligaments to make sure that they have not been disrupted.

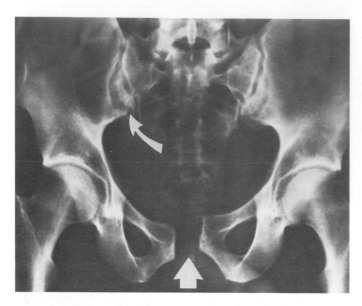

The pubic symphysis has been split open and the right sacro–iliac joint is widened.

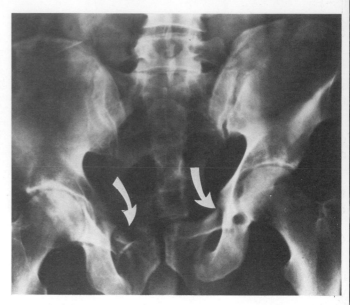

There are bilateral fractures of the pubic and conjoint rami.

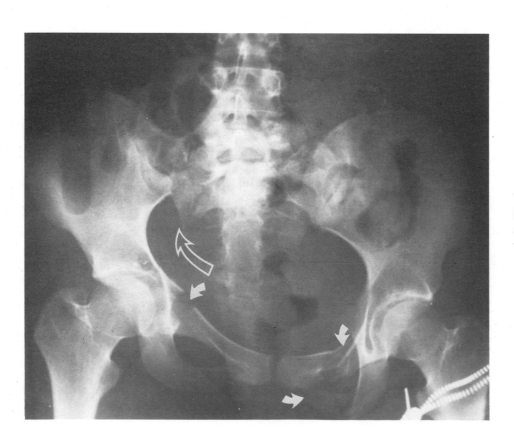

The right sacro-iliac joint is completely dislocated and there are fractures of the ischium and pubis.

## Pelvis *(continued)*

*Blood in the urine following trauma*

When there has been severe trauma, blood may appear in the urine (haematuria) owing to injury of the kidneys, ureters, bladder, or urethra. Always check the lower ribs and lumbar transverse processes both clinically and radiologically. If urinary-tract damage is suspected, an intravenous urogram will be necessary (pages 195-204).

*Urography*

Pelvic fractures may damage the bladder or urethra (more rarely, a ureter). The intravenous urogram will show the bladder on the 10- or 25-minute films. (Oblique films may be necessary to show the bladder clearly.)

If the bladder is compressed on both sides, this indicates a large haematoma in the pelvis. (The compression may occasionally be more on one side than the other.)

If there is leakage of contrast from the bladder into the pelvic cavity, either the ureter or the bladder has been damaged.

*Cystography*

If there is no clinical evidence of kidney damage and if there is a catheter already in the bladder, a cystogram will demonstrate damage. First empty the urine from the bladder, through the catheter. Then introduce 80 ml of diluted contrast solution. (Use 40 ml of standard IV contrast solution mixed with 40 ml of IV saline solution.) Take AP and oblique films of the patient.

If a male patient cannot void urine, the urethra may be damaged and the patient will need surgery. A urethrogram will define the damage. The technique is described on page 207, but when there has been trauma, first carefully introduce only 5 ml of contrast. Take the first film and check it for urethral or bladder leakage. If the urethra is normal, add a further 10 ml of contrast and re-X-ray. If extravasation is seen at any stage, STOP.

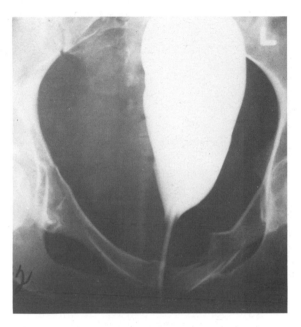

Bladder deformed by pelvic haematoma, larger on the right side.

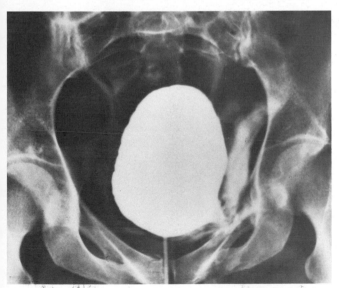

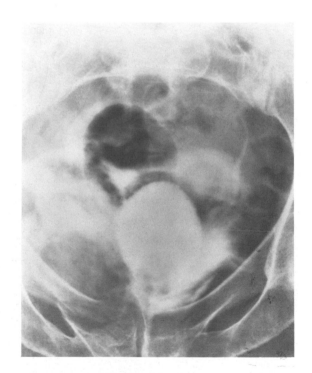

Two different patients with leakage of urine from rupture of the bladder due to pelvic fractures.

## Hip—Fractures and Dislocations

Dislocations of the hip result from severe trauma. The pelvis should be carefully checked to make sure there is no other injury to the acetabulum or pelvis.

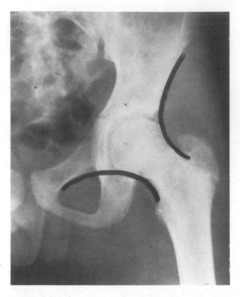

*Normal hip joint*

Check the two lines as shown on the radiograph. If the hip is dislocated, the lines will be interrupted. In a posterior dislocation the thigh is adducted; in an anterior dislocation (uncommon), the thigh is abducted.

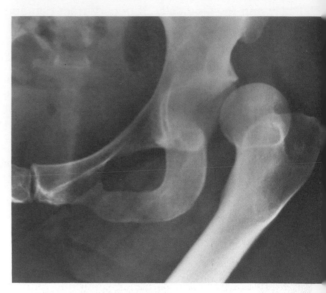

*Single posterior hip dislocation*

*Posterior hip dislocation with a fracture of posterior rim of the acetabulum*

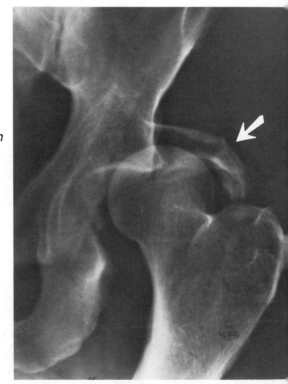

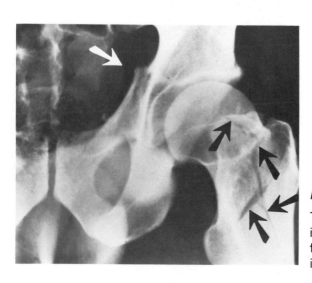

*Fracture of the acetabulum (white arrow)*

This type of fracture occurs when the femoral head is pushed into the hip joint. Note that there are also also fractures of the femoral neck and trochanters (black arrows). When the injury is severe, always look for more than one fracture.

## Hip—Fractures *(continued)*

Most hip fractures are easily seen, but difficulty may occur with subcapital fractures, particularly if these are slightly impacted with negligible displacement, as in the cases below.

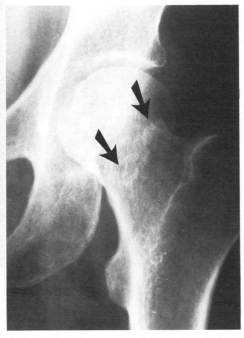

*Subcapital fracture with minimal deformity*

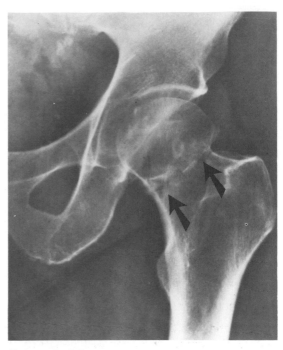

*Subcapital fracture*

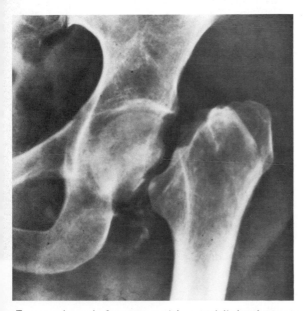

*Femoral neck fracture with established non-union*

The fracture gap is wide, the edges are smooth and dense. See page 87 for signs of non-union.

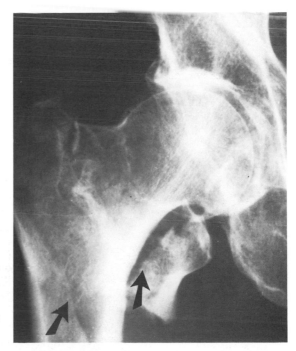

*Intertrochanteric fracture*

## Knee

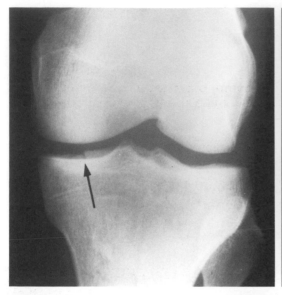

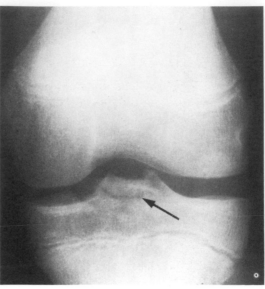

Fracture lines are arrowed.

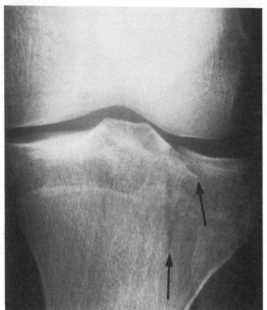

Fractures of the tibial plateau and tibial spines must be recognized.

When there is no depression of the fragment, open surgery to bone may not be needed. Do not forget that there will also be soft-tissue damage, particularly to the ligaments.

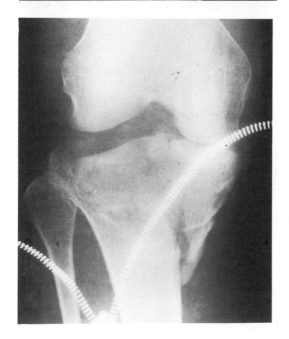

When the disruption is more severe, with greater irregularity of the articular surface, expert treatment will be needed to deal with bone and ligament damage.

**Knee** *(continued)*

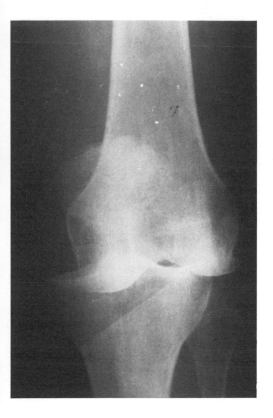

### Dislocated knee

The knee is not often dislocated, but when it is, the considerable force necessary to cause the dislocation will have severely damaged the ligaments.

The popliteal artery may have been damaged. The distal pulses must always be checked after reduction. Also check for distal sensation and movement to exclude nerve injury.

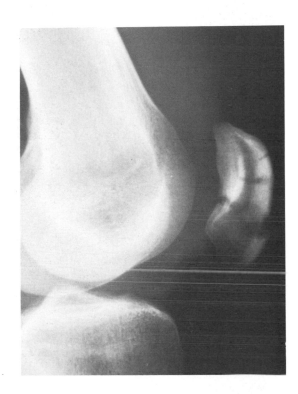

### Fractured patella

The patella (on the right) has been fractured as the result of direct trauma and it is in several fragments. Blood within the joint has displaced the bone anteriorly. In this comminuted fracture the fragments have not become widely separated. In transverse patellar fractures the fragments are often wide apart.

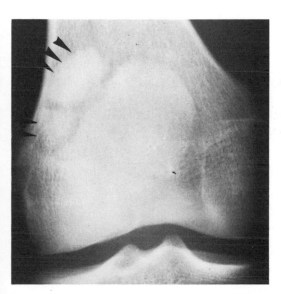

### Congenital variation of the patella (bipartite)

Sometimes there is a separate piece (ossicle) of bone at the upper and outer edge of the patella. This can be mistaken for a fracture but is a congenital variation. The other patella usually (but not always) looks the same. Careful clinical correlation will be necessary in such cases to decide whether the patella has been injured.

## Ankle

*Indications*

X-ray examination is needed ONLY when there is soft-tissue swelling and localized tenderness following acute injury. However, the absence of a fracture does not necessarily mean that the ankle does not need treatment. Radiographs only show bony damage and there may be severe ligamentous injury permitting dislocation (luxation), which is equally incapacitating.

Reduction of the dislocation precedes the reduction of the fractures and needs referral.

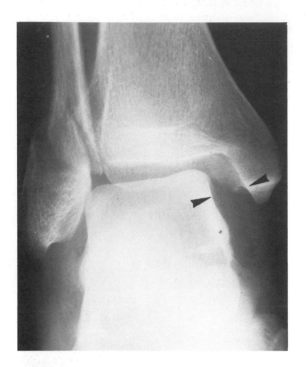

In this patient the space between the talus and the medial malleolus is very much widened (space between arrowheads). The lateral malleolus is laterally displaced. Such a situation indicates severe ligament damage, as well as the less important fracture of the fibula.

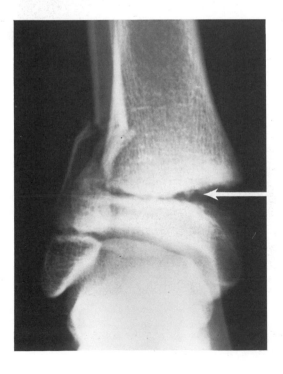

In this child, in addition to the fracture of the distal fibula, there is tilting of the ankle joint due to a fracture through the tibial growth plate, with a gap medially. This needs accurate repositioning.

> THE LATERAL VIEW OF THE ANKLE MUST BE CAREFULLY STUDIED TO EVALUATE THE EXTENT OF THE INJURY.

## Os Calcis

Fracture of the os calcis may be difficult to detect. As always, two views should be taken. Look particularly at the angle between the anterior and posterior parts of the os calcis in the lateral view (see *Normal*). In many calcaneal fractures due to a fall from a height, this angle is reduced or flattened.

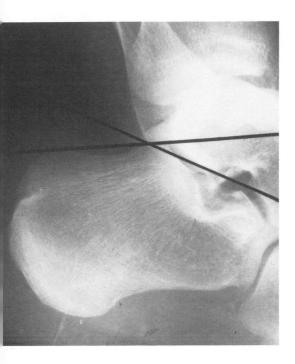

*Normal*

When normal, lines joining the upper edges of the posterior part and the middle part of the os calcis form an angle as shown. When a compression fracture deformity is present owing to crushing, the angle becomes smaller or may disappear (below left).

Os calcis fractures with deformity involving articular surfaces need referral for accurate reduction.

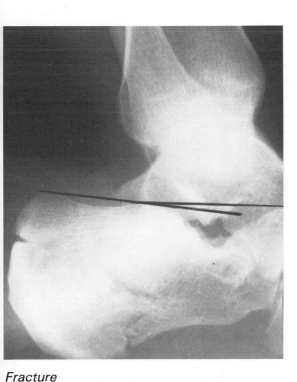

*Fracture*

Flattening of the angle due to fracture.

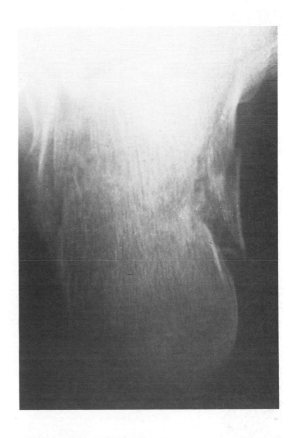

*Axial view*

This may show fragmentation, lateral or medial displacement, or involvement of the subtalar joint.

**Forefoot**

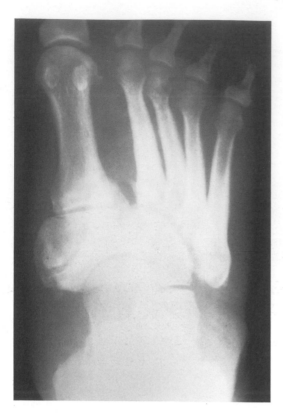
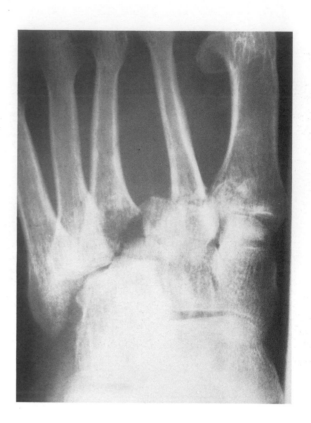

Fracture–dislocations of the forefoot at the metatarso-tarsal joints NEED CAREFUL EXAMINATION OF FILMS AS THEY MAY NOT BE OBVIOUS. This type of injury requires skilled treatment; it may be accompanied by damage to blood vessels.

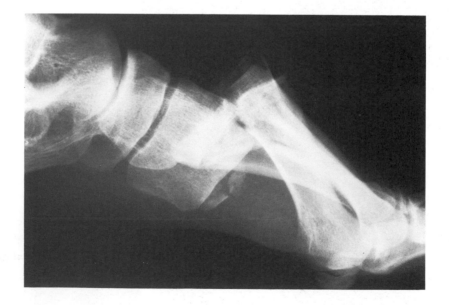

*Lateral view*

In this patient the fracture–dislocations are obvious, but this is not usually so.

**Forefoot** *(continued)*

## Metatarsal fractures

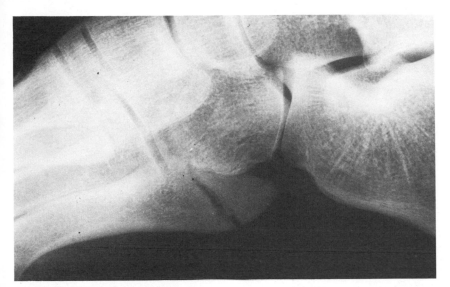

*Proximal transverse fracture*

### 5th metatarsal

The common avulsion fracture at the proximal end of the 5th metatarsal runs transversely across the bone. It must not be confused with the normal apophysis (during the growing period). The apophysis lies obliquely almost in the line of the metatarsal.

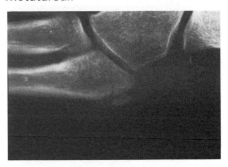

*Normal apophysis*

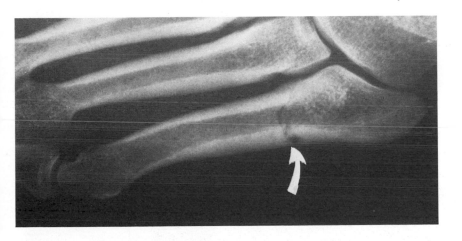

When the transverse fracture lies more distally (see left) it will need prolonged immobilization to allow healing.

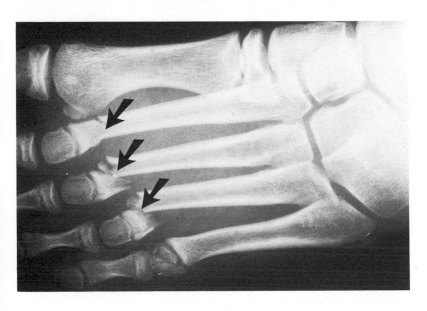

Fractures of the metatarsal necks are often multiple.

## BONE TUMOURS

Primary bone tumours are rare and it is very difficult to make an accurate radiological diagnosis of the type of tumour. It can also be difficult in some cases to distinguish tumour from infection.

### Benign Tumours

These are often painless, unless fractured. Size does not indicate whether a tumour is benign or malignant. Benign tumours have well-defined, clear edges. The cortex is usually unbroken, unless fractured.

There is seldom any periosteal reaction, unless fractured.

Such tumours are often best left alone: if doubtful about the diagnosis, refer the films for a specialist opinion.

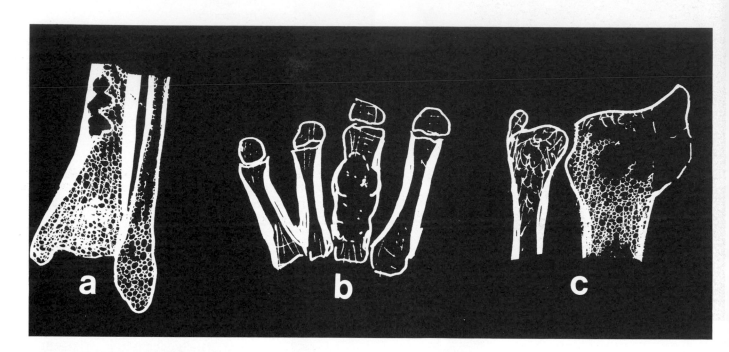

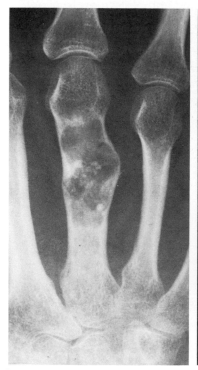

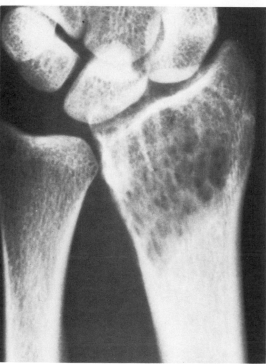

*(b) Enchondroma*

This is a common site for this tumour.

*(c) Giant cell tumour*

It may grow and make the bone much larger.

*(a) Fibrous cortical defect*

It arises in the cortex and extends to the medulla. Seen in the diaphyses of long bone, it is most common in the lower limb.

*(b) Enchondroma*

A common lesion in long bones, particularly the fingers. There is an area of bone expansion from within the medulla, with scalloped internal borders. Calcification may be present.

*(c) Giant cell tumour*

Occurs in young people, usually in their early twenties. An expanding lesion at the end of a long bone, with loss of trabeculae, ill-defined (internal) edges and thin septa crossing the lesion. Such tumours can easily fracture as they grow larger.

## Malignant Tumours

Primary bone tumours are very rare; they require expert interpretation.
They are usually single.
Metastatic bone tumours are more common; they are often multiple.
Malignant tumours (primary or secondary) may destroy bone; form new bone around the tumour; increase or decrease the density of the bone; they are ill-defined and invasive; they are often accompanied by a mass and may be painful.

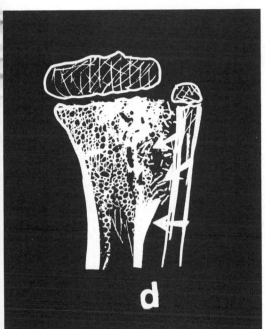

destroyed
bone spicules

periosteal
reaction

### Osteogenic sarcoma

A disease of children and young adults. There are many varieties. Depicted here is a representation of a classic case with ill-defined destruction of cortex and trabeculae, new bone sclerosis endosteally, and bone spicules extending into a soft-tissue mass. At the lower edge there is a triangular area of periosteal new bone formation.

### Other malignant bone tumours

These are destructive and seldom show so much spiculation. But the diagnosis is difficult. SEND THE FILMS AND FULL CLINICAL DETAILS (and a PA chest film) for a specialist opinion. DO NOT DELAY.

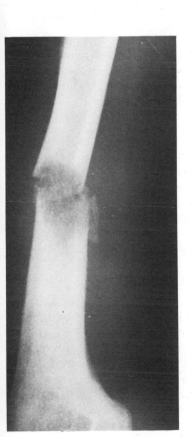

### Metastases

These can occur in any bone, anywhere. They are usually (but not always) locally painful. They are usually destructive (lytic) and fractures may result when the bone is weakened. Occasionally they are dense (particularly when the primary tumour is in the prostate or the female breast). There is seldom much periosteal new bone (as compared with primary bone tumours). Most important, they are almost always multiple, occurring in different bones. It is seldom possible to recognize the primary from which the metastases arise. They all look much the same.

## BONE INFECTION (OSTEOMYELITIS)

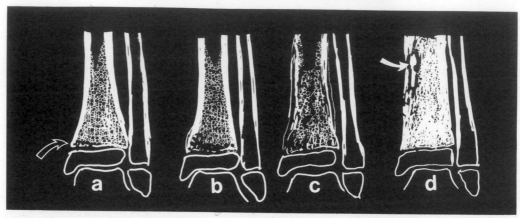

(1) IN EARLY STAGES (10–14 days) THERE ARE NO X-RAY CHANGES: the diagnosis must be made clinically (local pain, fever, leukocytosis) aided by blood culture.

(2) Childhood osteomyelitis progresses through four stages:

(a) Initially there is an area of bone destruction near the metaphysis.
(b) In a few days this extends into the shaft and transversely, attacks the adjacent cortex and elevates the periosteum.
(c) As the disorder progresses there is permeative destruction (osteoporosis), more cortical destruction, and obvious periosteal new bone parallelling the original cortex.
(d) In the late stage a thick periosteal envelope develops, with sclerosis, expanded bone, and sequestrum (arrowed) that may need surgical removal.

(3) Soft-tissue infection can spread into bone and cause local osteomyelitis.

(4) Soft-tissue infection near bone may also cause changes in the bone without actual bone infection. There may be increased or decreased bone density.

Do not forget that these appearances may be due to sickle-cell disease.

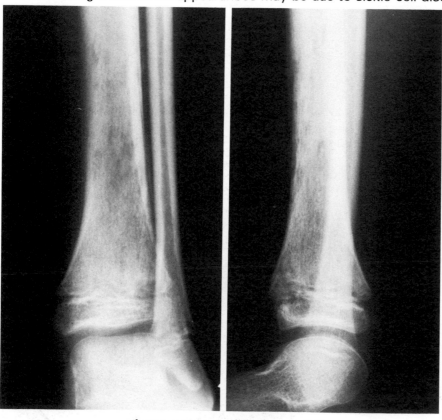

*Acute osteomyelitis (stage (b))*

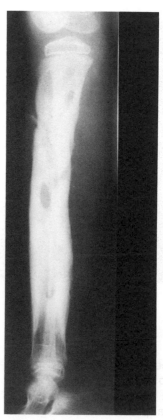

*Chronic osteomyelitis (stage (d))*

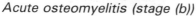

# ARTHRITIS

Pain in a joint can be due to numerous causes. If of recent onset, particularly in an acute process accompanied by fever, X-ray changes may be seen only after two to three weeks. If a septic arthritis is suspected, treat appropriately and do not wait until X-ray changes have developed.

More chronic joint pains can be due to a variety of conditions. We have chosen the painful hip for illustrative purposes, but the same appearance may be seen in any joint.

## Osteoarthritis

In this process the joint space narrows, usually at the site of maximum weight-bearing, sclerosis (increase in whiteness) develops around the affected area, and marginal bony protuberances and cysts form. A normal hip (a) and progressive changes are illustrated diagrammatically and in radiographs.

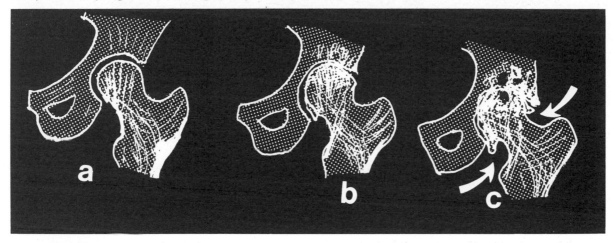

(a) Normal hip.
(b) Loss of clear joint space superiorly and sclerosis beneath articular surfaces.
(c) Osteophyte formation (arrowed), total loss of joint space, subarticular cysts, and increasing sclerosis.

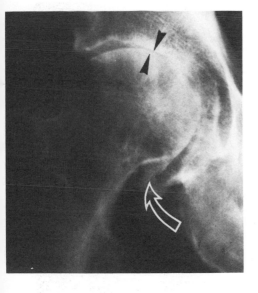

Osteoarthritic hip at stage (b) with loss of joint space (black arrows) and marginal osteophyte (hollow arrow). Some sclerosis and cyst-like lesions are beginning to appear.

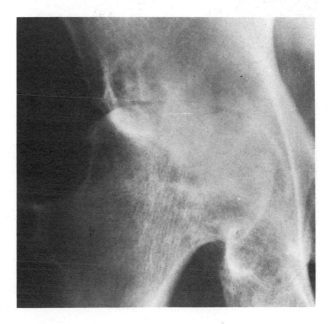

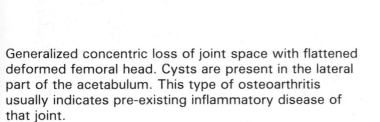

Generalized concentric loss of joint space with flattened deformed femoral head. Cysts are present in the lateral part of the acetabulum. This type of osteoarthritis usually indicates pre-existing inflammatory disease of that joint.

## Tuberculous Arthritis

This form of infection usually involves only one joint. The changes slowly progress so that the joint loses its well-defined margins as bone is destroyed. The diagram and radiographs illustrate the process.

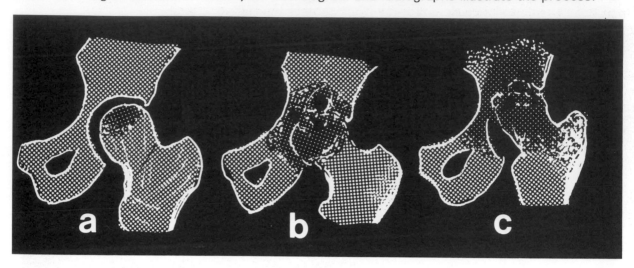

(*a*) Initially the only evidence of tuberculosis may be widening of the joint space from effusion and peri-articular osteoporosis.

(*b*) As the infection develops, osteoporosis spreads; foci of bone destruction may appear in the femoral head and acetabulum, and the white line subchondral bone plate is destroyed.

(*c*) With progressive destruction, the femoral head migrates superiorly and the joint space disappears.

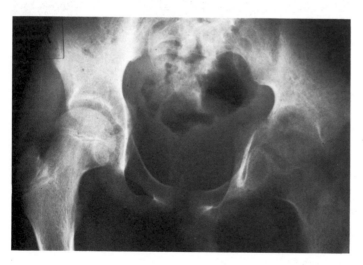

*Early-stage synovial TB of the left hip*

Note loss of bone density on the affected left side.

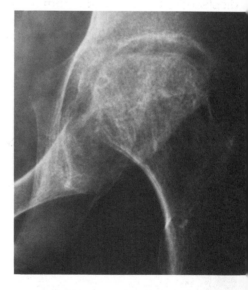

*Later-stage infection*

As the tuberculous infection continues, osteoporosis is pronounced, the joint space widens, and the acetabulum becomes excavated allowing the femoral head to move upwards.

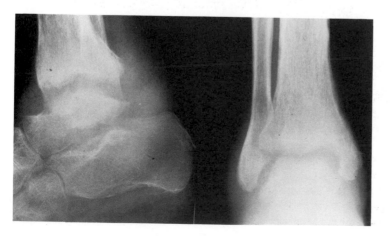

*Tuberculous arthritis of the ankle*

In this advanced case, the normal well-defined articular contours of the tibia and talus have disappeared.

## Pain in the Hip

Before requesting the X-ray examination, check the spine and the knees clinically. Pain in the hip may be due to an abnormal gait, or either spinal or hip pathology.

There are many different causes of pain in the hip other than acute trauma.

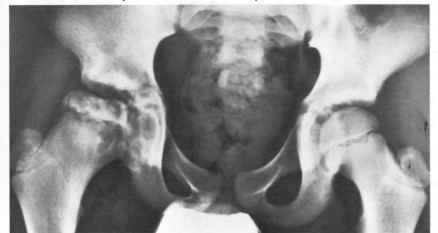

*Perthes' disease of the right hip*

Childhood: avascular necrosis (Perthes' disease) causes deformity of the femoral head which becomes more dense than usual (whiter) and appears to fragment.
Eventually the femoral neck will become widened and cystic. This may take two years, with intermittent pain-free periods, which do not mean that the process has stopped.

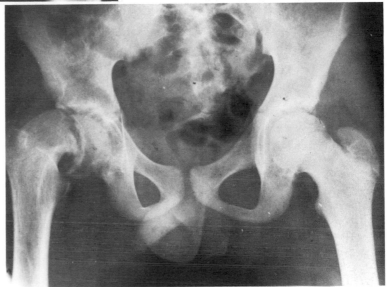

*Displaced femoral epiphysis*

Childhood: the femoral epiphysis may be displaced with loss of the normal round femoral head and with the epiphysis sliding off like a cap, as in the right hip.

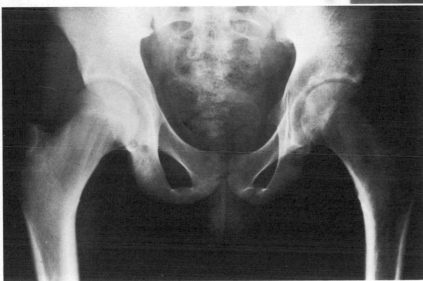

*Joint infection (infective arthritis)*

At any age, joint infection may cause pain. The earliest X-ray findings can be difficult to recognize. There is haziness around the joint. Later the bones become osteoporotic (less dense, less white, and more grey in appearance). The difference between the normal and the abnormal joint is very helpful. The left side is affected in this instance. All infections (acute pyogenic, tuberculous, etc.) look the same radiologically. Tuberculosis is usually only slowly progressive; other infections may change more rapidly.

## Rheumatoid Arthritis

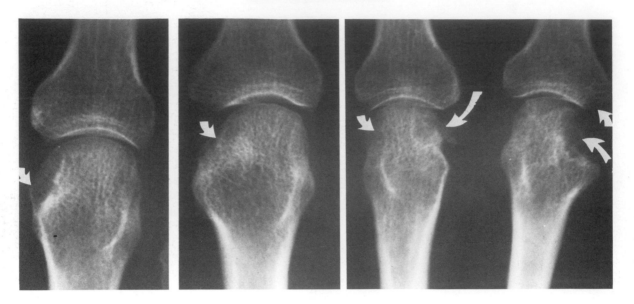

Progressive stages in erosions from rheumatoid arthritis affecting metacarpo-phalangeal joints. The arrows indicate the sites involved in these different patients. The earliest change is a barely visible break in the subchondral white line. As the disease progresses, larger areas are involved until significant wedges of bone have disappeared.

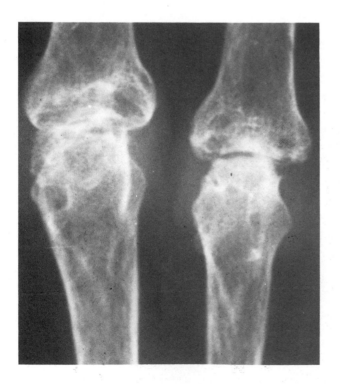

With even more advanced erosive destruction, the excavation is more pronounced and may involve both sides of a joint.

### Rheumatoid Arthritis *(continued)*

The ligaments are also involved, so that they become stretched and allow medial subluxation of the fingers.

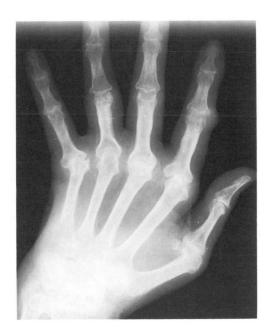

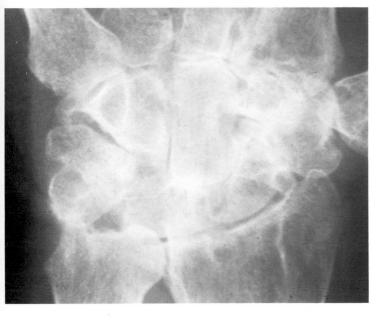

Erosive polyarthropathy often affects the wrist joint, leading to osteoporosis and loss of joint space. Ultimately the individual carpal bones may fuse.

### Gout

At the time of the early painful attacks of gout, it is unlikely that the bones will show any changes. Later, well-defined rounded cyst-like marginal bone defects may appear, particularly at the first metatarsophalangeal joint. Frequently soft-tissue swelling due to tophi can be seen medially (white arrows). (These findings are not entirely specific for gout.)

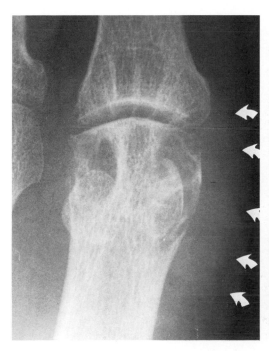
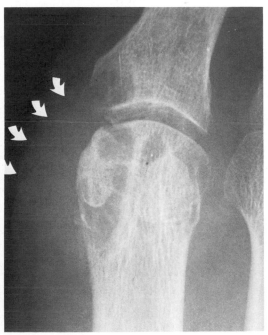

# SKULL X-RAYS

# THE SKULL

DOUBLE PAGE
FOLD-OUT

Clinical Examination

MUST

PRECEDE

X-Ray Examination

If the skull views are not correctly positioned the appearances can be misleading.

When using the
following pages,
keep this open to help
to identify the anatomy
of the skull.

## CHECK POSITION

(1) In the lateral view the temporomandibular joints must be superimposed.
(2) The clinoid processes must be symmetrical.
(3) In the frontal views the sagittal suture must be in the midline and the outline of the skull symmetrical.

## NORMAL SKULL
### Landmarks
anterior fontanelle—closes at 24 months

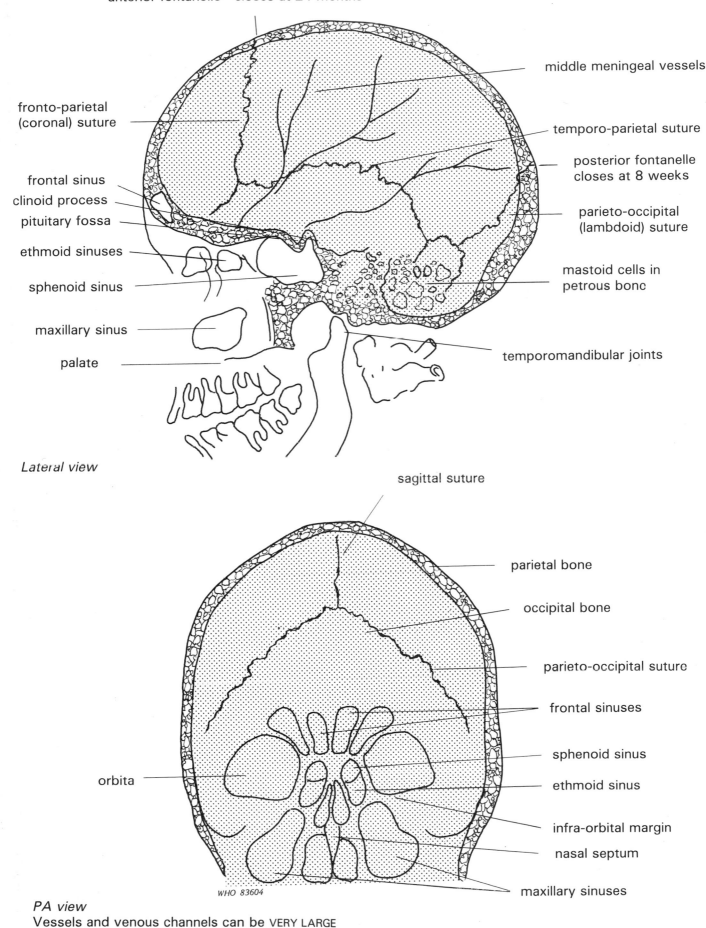

fronto-parietal (coronal) suture

frontal sinus
clinoid process
pituitary fossa
ethmoid sinuses
sphenoid sinus

maxillary sinus

palate

middle meningeal vessels

temporo-parietal suture

posterior fontanelle closes at 8 weeks

parieto-occipital (lambdoid) suture

mastoid cells in petrous bone

temporomandibular joints

*Lateral view*

sagittal suture

parietal bone

occipital bone

parieto-occipital suture

frontal sinuses

sphenoid sinus

ethmoid sinus

infra-orbital margin

nasal septum

maxillary sinuses

orbita

WHO 83604

*PA view*
Vessels and venous channels can be VERY LARGE

# THE SKULL

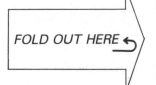

*FOLD OUT HERE*

Clinical Examination

MUST

PRECEDE

X-Ray Examination

# INDICATIONS FOR SKULL X-RAYS

A careful clinical examination is necessary before X-raying the skull. This will help to obtain the correct X-ray films and correlate the clinical and radiological findings. The skull is very difficult to interpret radiologically; let the X-rays help but NOT REPLACE your clinical judgement.

Indications for X-rays include:

(1) *Trauma.* SEVERE head injury in adults, especially with prolonged loss of consciousness or when there is clinical evidence of a depressed fracture, is a clear indication for X-rays (page 134).

    (a) *Mild trauma.* If the patient has not lost consciousness or has only been unconscious briefly, and if the clinical examination is normal, it is probable that skull X-rays will not alter your treatment. Clinical signs will be far more important (loss of consciousness, change in pulse or respiration, fits, double vision, etc.).

    (b) *Trauma in children.* It is usually easy to detect a depressed fracture in a child by clinical examination and skull X-rays are then necessary to show the extent of the injury and the treatment needed. Mild head injury with normal clinical examination is NOT an indication for X-rays because it is unlikely that treatment will be altered. Most skull X-rays in children following trauma are unhelpful; careful clinical observation is more important.

(2) *Bleeding from the ears* or cerebrospinal fluid leaking from the ears or nose after trauma almost always means a fracture of the base of the skull. This is very difficult to recognize on X-rays. A lateral view taken with the patient lying supine may show blood in the sphenoid sinus or air within the skull (page 135).

(3) *A local bulge (or dent)* in the skull. X-rays may help in the diagnosis provided the bulge is fixed on clinical examination, and not mobile (i.e., not only in the scalp). If the bulge is soft, an X-ray of that area will help to exclude an underlying skull defect (infection, tumour, etc.).

(4) *Persistent headache.* X-rays seldom provide much useful information UNLESS there are clinical signs— e.g., neurological abnormality, raised intracranial pressure (optical signs), or blindness. If the patient is known to have a primary malignant tumour elsewhere, a lateral skull X-ray may help to show skull metastases.

(5) *Earache.* Clinical examination is better than X-rays unless you are an expert on mastoid X-rays. Routine skull films are seldom helpful when mastoiditis is suspected.

(6) *Metastases* or general disease, such as Paget's disease. A lateral view of the skull may help in the diagnosis. Additional views are unhelpful.

---

SKULL X-RAYS ARE SELDOM HELPFUL IN MOST CASES OF DISEASE OF THE CENTRAL NERVOUS SYSTEM, UNLESS THERE IS CLEAR EVIDENCE OF A CRANIAL NERVE ABNORMALITY OR CLINICAL EVIDENCE OF RAISED INTRACRANIAL PRESSURE.

# NORMAL SKULL

## Search Pattern, Lateral Skull

Look at the shape of the whole skull. Is there any area which bulges outwards or is dented inwards?

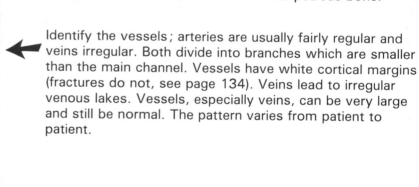

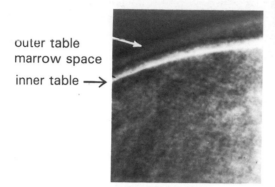

outer table
marrow space
inner table →

Follow the lines of the inner and outer tables all around the skull vault.

Look at the density of the skull. There are always areas which are less dense at the front and the back. The base of the skull is white because of the petrous bone.

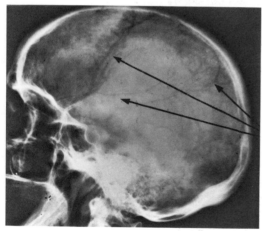

Identify the vessels; arteries are usually fairly regular and veins irregular. Both divide into branches which are smaller than the main channel. Vessels have white cortical margins (fractures do not, see page 134). Veins lead to irregular venous lakes. Vessels, especially veins, can be very large and still be normal. The pattern varies from patient to patient.

When possible look at the teeth; in children there will be a translucent (dark) area around the roots while they are growing. In adults such an area usually means an abscess or, if there are several little holes, osteomyelitis or occasionally lymphoma.

The dense white shadows are dental fillings.

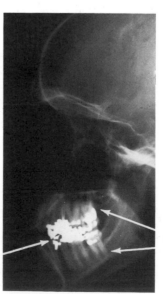

abscess (adult patient)

dental roots

## Search Pattern, Lateral Skull *(continued)*

Then identify the pituitary fossa on the base of the skull in front of the white petrous bone. Below it is the translucent (dark) sphenoid sinus.

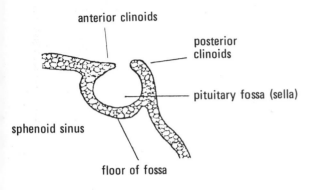

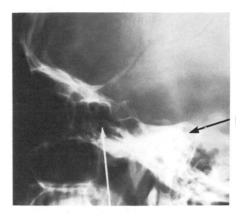

sphenoid sinus

**Frontal (AP) Projection**
*Quality control*

The orbits must be symmetrical, with the nasal bones in the centre of the film. The mandible should appear equal on both sides.
The dense white petrous bones should be across the lower part of the orbits.

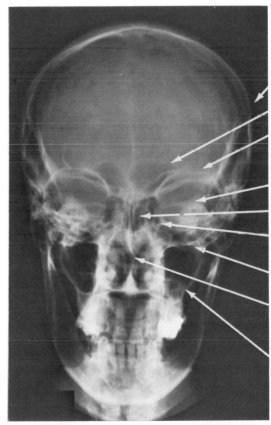

temporo-parietal suture

frontal sinus

supra-orbital ridge

orbit

sphenoid sinus

ethmoid sinus

infra-orbital ridge

nasal septum

maxillary antrum

*Search pattern*

Look at the shape of the skull. Is there any part which bulges outwards or is dented inwards? Follow the white line of the cortex from one side over the top of the skull to the other side. Is there any area of different density? (The lateral aspects along the temporal bones always seem more translucent.) Identify the supra-orbital ridges and the infra-orbital margins.

Look for the frontal sinus. This is often asymmetrical in shape and uneven in density. The ethmoid and sphenoid sinuses are on either side of the nose. The maxillary antra, below the orbit, should be of equal translucency.

# SKULL FRACTURES

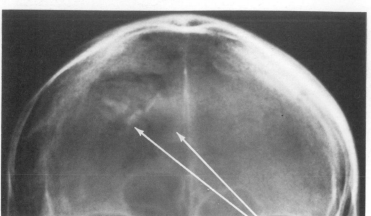

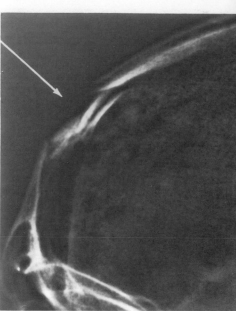

Fractures are seen as black lines, but where there is an overlap of the fragments the lines will be white.

*Depressed fractures of the right frontal bone*

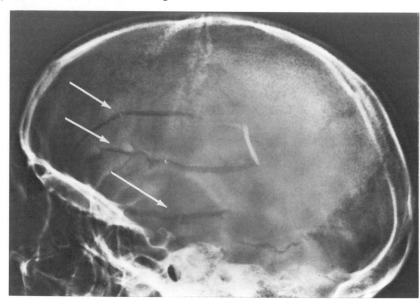

*Linear fractures*              *Lateral vie*

These must be differentiated from vessels. Fractures vary in calibre, they seldom branch, have no white margin, and may be anywhere. Vessels must be in the correct anatomical direction, have white margins and branch to smaller vessels. The patient's clinical condition and soft-tissue swelling are very helpful indicators.

A branching vessel with white margins.

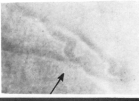

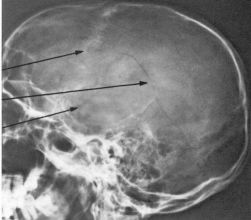

sutures

fractures

vessel

*Semi-axial (Towne's) projection*

When the posterior part of the skull, the occiput, is injured you must have this Towne's projection (left).

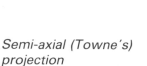

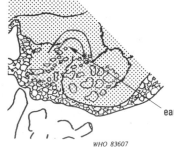

ear

*WHO 83607*

Do not forget that the shadow of the ear (the pinna) can look like a fracture or intracerebral calcification.

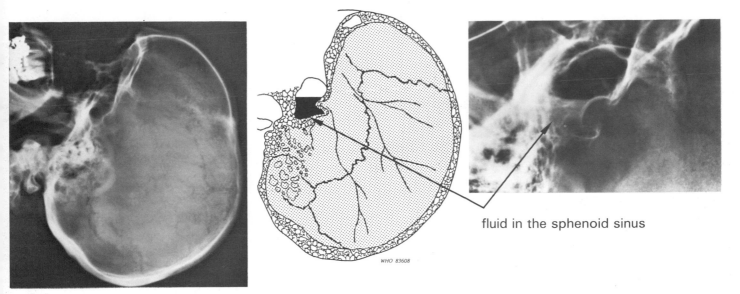

fluid in the sphenoid sinus

If you suspect a fracture at the base of the skull, take a cross-table lateral view with the head in the position shown above. You may see fluid (blood or cerebrospinal fluid) in the sphenoid sinus. Unless the patient has severe sinusitis, this can only be due to a fracture at the base of the skull.

Fractures of the nasal sinuses may allow air to escape into the orbits, especially when the patient blows his nose. This causes orbital emphysema, and the air shows as a black line across the roof of the orbit if the X-ray is taken with the patient sitting up.

A small amount of air in the right orbit. There is more in the left orbit.

Do not mistake the gap between the eyelids for air. This will be in the middle of the orbit; air will be at the top.

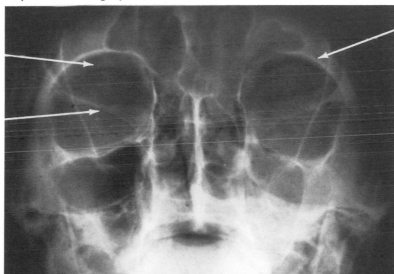

Air in the left orbit following facial trauma. Infection may follow this type of injury. It is seldom possible to recognize the actual fracture, but if there is air in the orbit, there must be an injury.

*Fractured mandible*

Take sinus views and a PA view of the skull. Add obliques if necessary. Mandibular fractures are often bilateral; look carefully for the second injury and check clinically. The parts of the mandible near the temporo-mandibular joint and at the angle are where fractures are often missed radiologically.

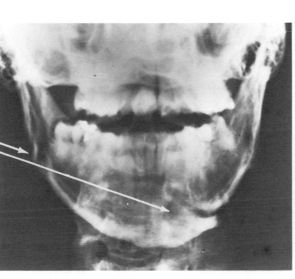

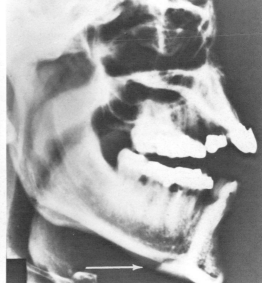

## FACIAL TRAUMA

right orbit    nose    left orbit

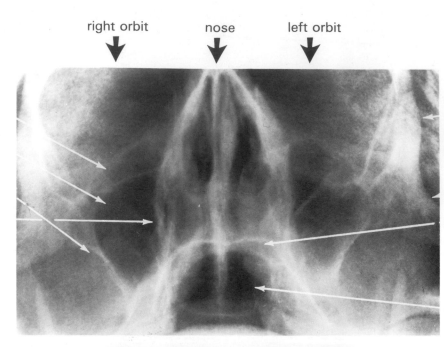

**The Normal**

orbital floor

right antrum

lateral wall of
antrum

medial wall of
antrum

lateral wall of the
orbit (the orbital
process of the
maxilla)

zygoma

palate

sphenoid sinus

**Injured Left Face**

*Checklist uninjured side*

Lateral wall of orbit: intact.
Floor of orbit: intact.
Right antrum: clear.
Lateral wall of antrum: intact.
Mandible: intact.

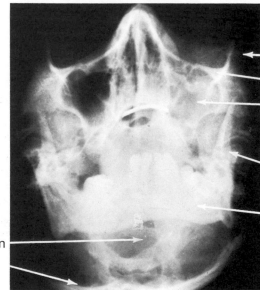

foramen magnum
base of skull

*Checklist injured side*

Lateral wall of orbit: intact.

Floor of orbit: fractured

Left antrum: opaque owing
to blood and soft-tissue
swelling.

Mandible: ascending ramus
intact.

Mandible: body intact.

> SINGLE FRACTURES OF THE
> ORBIT ARE UNUSUAL.

**Injured Right Face**

*Checklist injured side*

Supra-orbital margin: intact.

Lateral wall of orbit: intact.

Floor of orbit: fractured.

Antrum: opaque.
Lateral wall of antrum:
fractured.
    Zygoma: intact.

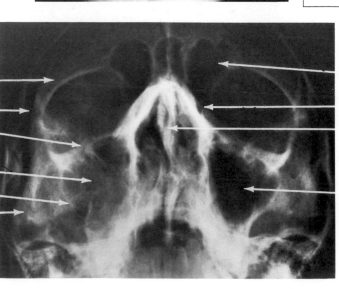

*Checklist uninjured side*

Frontal sinuses: clear.

Nasal bones: intact.

Septum displaced: this
is common and seldom
traumatic.

Left antrum: clear, all
margins intact.

## Injured Right Face

*Checklist*

Supra-orbital margin: intact.

Lateral wall of orbit: intact.

Floor of orbit: fractured and depressed.

Right antrum: opaque owing to blood in antrum and soft-tissue swelling.

Lateral wall of antrum: intact.

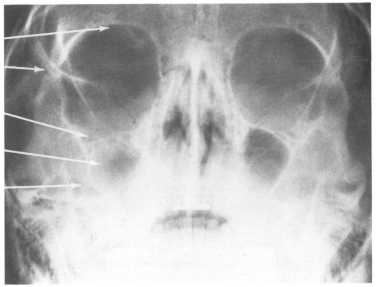

Nasal septum and nasal bones: intact.

## Injured Left Face

*Right side:*

Right supra-orbital margin fractured.

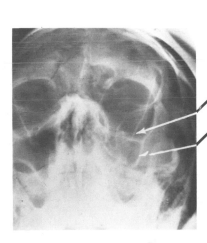

*Checklist: injured side*

Left supra-orbital margin: intact.
Left lateral orbital margin: intact.
Floor of orbit: fractured and depressed.
Antrum: opaque owing to blood and soft-tissue swelling.
Zygoma: intact.
Nasal bones: fractured and displaced.
Lateral wall of antrum: superimposed on petrous bone. Not clearly seen.

*Right side:* appears intact (fracture not visible).

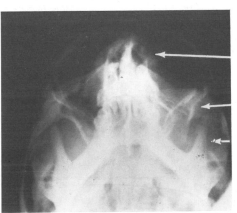

*Same patient: angle of X-ray increased (head tilted another 10°).*
Nasal bones: fractured and displaced.

Lateral wall of antrum: fractured inwards.

Ascending ramus of mandible: intact.
Zygoma: intact.

Mandible intact.

# PITUITARY FOSSA (SELLA TURCICA)

An important landmark at the base of the skull.

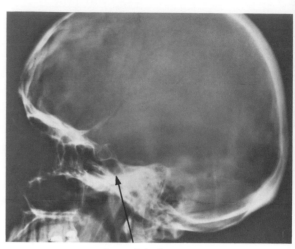

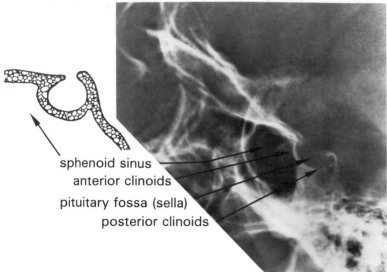

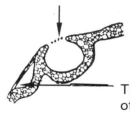

sphenoid sinus
anterior clinoids
pituitary fossa (sella)
posterior clinoids

sphenoid sinus

The pituitary fossa can be completely or partially bridged.

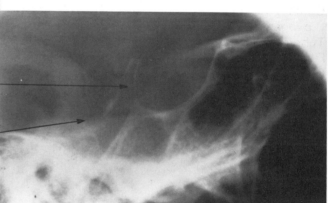

The petro-clinoid ligament often calcifies. Neither is clinically significant.

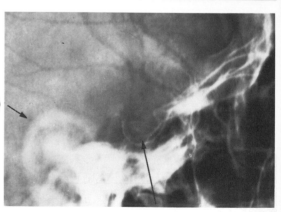

The ear (pinna)

The clinoids may partially or completely disappear for two reasons: raised intracranial pressure or local pituitary disease. The sella can be enlarged by a pituitary tumour (adenoma) or by raised intracranial pressure (examine the optic fundus). When enlarged, the floor thins.

Calcification over this enlarged fossa is due to the carotid artery. It could also be a pituitary tumour.

If the floor of the fossa is eroded or destroyed (arrow), this is usually due to a malignant tumour in the fossa or spreading from below. This does not happen when the fossa is enlarged by raised intracranial pressure, which can cause thinning but not erosion.

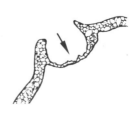

# LYTIC DEFECTS IN SKULL

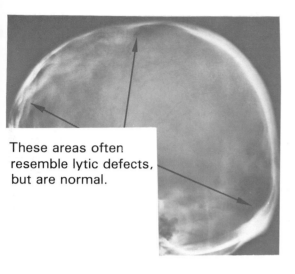

These areas often resemble lytic defects, but are normal.

The lytic defect of a metastasis from a carcinoma of the breast.

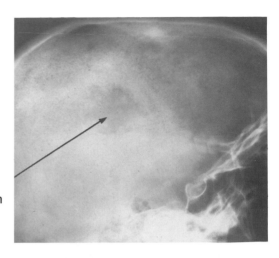

## Solitary Lytic Defect

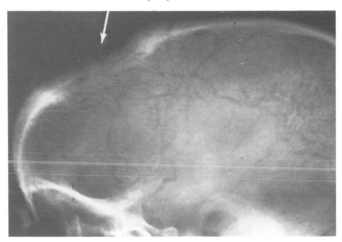

Osteomyelitis due to
  pyogenic organisms.
Tuberculosis.
Fungus.
Gumma (syphilis).
Hydatid disease (usually
  smooth outline).
Eosinophilic granuloma.
Histiocytosis.

Malignant origin.
Metastases from any
  primary neoplasm.
Tumour of the scalp.
Myeloma (usually mul-
  tiple).

*Remember* to exclude previous surgery (burr hole) and trauma.

A defect with:

— Smooth edges; usually a benign tumour, but may be infection or a surgical burr hole.
— Smooth dense edges; chronic infection or a slowly growing tumour or hydatid.
— Rough ill-defined edges; malignant or acute infection.
— Buttonhole appearance; usually infection, especially tuberculosis, syphilis, fungus; eosinophilic granuloma.

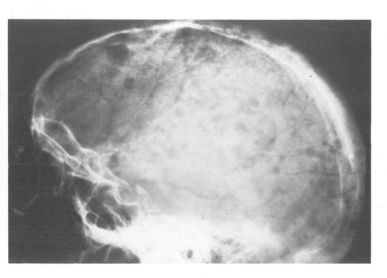

## Multiple Lytic Defects

— Metastases from any primary neoplasm.
— Multiple myeloma.
— Occasionally, syphilis, fungus, or other
  infections.

# DENSE AREAS IN SKULL

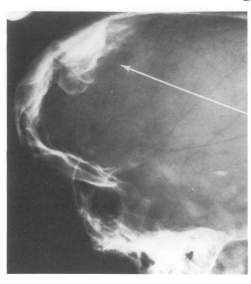

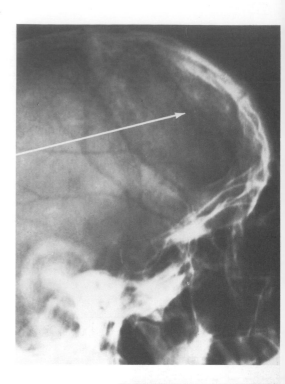

*Hyperostosis frontalis*

In the frontal area, increased density and calcification of the meninges can occur normally with aging (hyperostosis frontalis). It has no significance.

## Meningioma

Smooth and dense bone inside any part of the skull may be due to meningioma. In the early stages there may be very few central nervous system signs; headache is a warning sign when it becomes persistent.

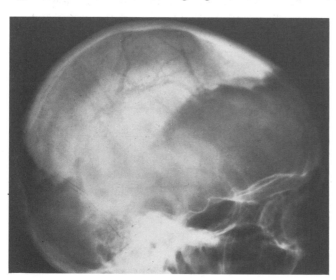

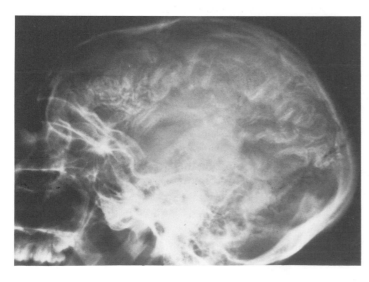

*Osteoporosis circumscripta*

Bones may appear dense because other nearby bones are less dense. The parietal bone in this case is normal, the frontal and occipital bones are hypertranslucent owing to early Paget's disease (see facing page). This may be localized or extensive, as in the case shown, but invariably progresses to typical Paget's disease.

*Calcification in the brain*

This has many causes (see also facing page). When it is linear, the common causes are a glioma, arteriovenous aneurysm, haemangioma or (as in this case) Sturge-Weber syndrome.
Do not forget that the ear (the pinna) can look like a ring of increased density (see pages 134, 138).

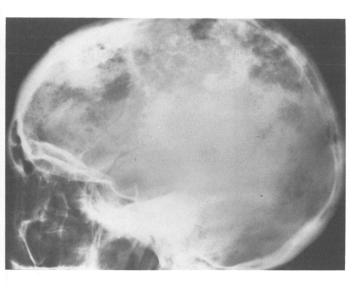

## Infection

Patchy densities and translucent areas usually mean infection, in this case syphilis. Malignant disease (metastases), fungus infection (mycetoma), and myeloma can all resemble this pattern.

AS WITH ALL RADIOLOGICAL FINDINGS, CORRELATE CLINICALLY.

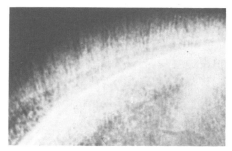

*Haemolytic disorder*

## Paget's disease

Patchy round densities (see left) have two common causes; metastases (especially from breast or prostate) or Paget's disease. In Paget's disease the skull vault is always thickened, as in this patient. In metastases there is never generalized thickening, but sometimes some local thickening. Haemolytic disorder also causes expansion of the outer table. If in doubt, X-ray the chest and pelvis to look for metastases in the lungs or other evidence of Paget's disease.

## Calcification in the brain

### Tuberculomas

This can be imitated by dirt or tightly woven hair.
*Speckled calcification.* Glioma or other tumour.
*Multiple small nodules.* Cysticercosis. Tuberous sclerosis.
*Irregular or cystic calcification.* Tuberculoma, hydatid disease.
*Smooth dense calcification.* Haematoma, hydatid disease, meningioma.

Remember that the pineal and choroid plexuses will also calcify normally. This is not significant unless they are displaced.

Pinna.

**SINUSES**

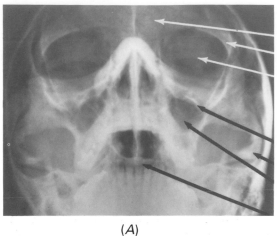

(A)

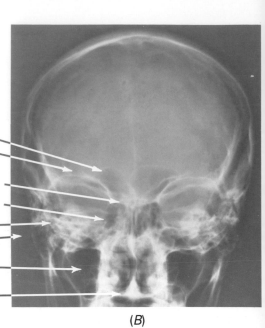

frontal sinus
orbital ridge
eyelid across orbit
sphenoid sinus
ethmoid sinus
infra-orbital ridge
zygoma
maxillary sinus
palate

(B)

## Sinus X-Rays

*Indications*

Local pain, swelling or trauma. Foul nasal discharge.

Sinuses always need at least two projections, (A) and (B).

*Search pattern—frontal views*

Identify the orbits, then the maxillary antra below each orbit; the frontal sinuses above and between the orbits; then the ethmoids and sphenoids as shown above ((A) and (B)).

*Lateral view*

Identify the pituitary fossa (1).
Below this is the sphenoid (2).
In front of the sphenoid are the ethmoids (3).
Below the ethmoids are the maxillary antra (4).
Above the antra are the orbits, and above them are frontal sinuses (5) at the front of the skull. Inspect each carefully, looking at the density and the outline of the sinus. The frontal sinuses are often differently shaped on each side.

*Common abnormalities seen in the sinuses (erect PA view)*

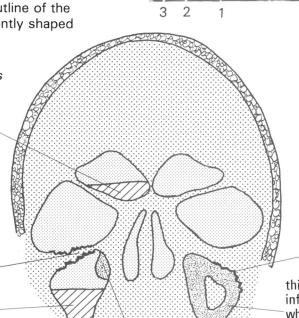

fluid in
frontal sinus

fracture of
orbital margin

fluid in
maxillary sinus

destroyed or widene[d]
wall of sinus due to
neoplasm

thick mucosa due to
infection (may fill
whole sinus)

mucosal polyp
(infection)

WHO 83610

# THE SKULL: DIFFERENTIAL DIAGNOSIS

## Closure of Sutures and Fontanelles

(1) Anterior fontanelle closes at any date up to 24 months.
(2) Posterior fontanelle usually closes within 2 or 3 months.
(3) The frontal parietal suture (the coronal suture) should be completely fused at the age of 30 years.
(4) The parietal occipital suture (the lambdoid suture) should be completely fused by the age of 30 years.
(5) The temporal parietal suture (the squamosal suture) should be completely fused by the age of 20–30 years.

ALL THESE DATES AND OTHER INFORMATION REPRESENT ACCEPTED "NORMALS". HOWEVER, THERE IS WIDE VARIATION AMONG INDIVIDUALS.

## Causes of a Large Head

*In children:*

(1) Hydrocephalus.
(2) Brain tumour.
(3) Hydatid disease.
(4) Meningitis with cerebral oedema (including tuberculosis).
(5) Achondroplasia (with short legs and arms).
(6) Subdural haematoma.

*In adults:*

(1) Paget's disease.
(2) Fibrous dysplasia.
(3) Acromegaly.

## Causes of a Small Head

*In children:*

(1) Congenital: idiopathic small brain, Down's syndrome.
(2) Craniostenosis (with beaten-copper appearance and sutures closed early).
(3) Tuberous sclerosis (with scattered small intracranial calcifications).
(4) Prenatal infections: toxoplasmosis, rubella, herpes, syphilis.

*In adults:*

Almost always the result of childhood disease.

# SPINAL X-RAYS

# SPINAL X-RAYS

## SEARCH PATTERN

Look at each part of the spine in the same way; the sequence is the same for the cervical, thoracic, and lumbar regions.

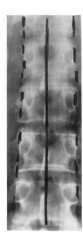

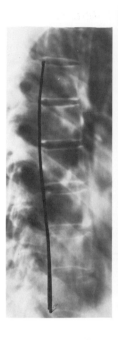

### AP view

Look at the alignment. At all levels the vertebrae should be in a straight line or only slightly curved.

### Lateral projection

Look at the posterior part of the vertebral bodies. The curve should be smooth without any abrupt step or change in direction.

### AP view

Next look at the shape of each vertebral body. This must be done very carefully. There are no "short-cuts". The transverse processes and the pedicles (the white oval) are visible (1).

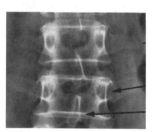

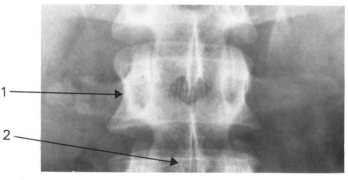

The spinous processes (2) will vary slightly in shape and angulation. Then look at the disc spaces. In the cervical and lumbar areas look for the paravertebral joints, which are not always easily seen.

### Lateral projection

Follow the same routine: look at EACH vertebral body. In each region of the spine they should be about the same size and shape. Also look at each intervertebral space. These should also be about the same width at each level. If the spaces seem to be narrowed, look carefully at the surrounding vertebral bodies for any change in shape or density. Then look at the density inside each vertebra very carefully. (Overlying bowel gas may resemble a lucency. Correlate with the AP view of the same vertebra.)

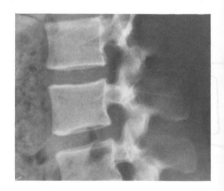

THE NORMAL SPINE HAS FORWARD CURVATURE IN THE CERVICAL AREA, BACKWARD (KYPHOTIC) CURVATURE IN THE THORACIC AREA, AND FORWARD (LORDOTIC) CURVATURE IN THE LUMBAR AREA. IF ANY PART OF THE SPINE IS STRAIGHT OR HAS A REVERSE CURVATURE, SEEK THE CAUSE.

# NORMAL CERVICAL SPINE

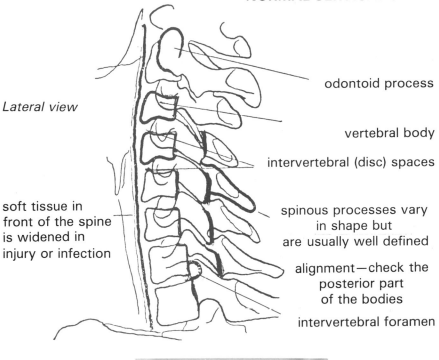

*Lateral view*

odontoid process

vertebral body

intervertebral (disc) spaces

spinous processes vary
in shape but
are usually well defined

alignment—check the
posterior part
of the bodies

intervertebral foramen

soft tissue in
front of the spine
is widened in
injury or infection

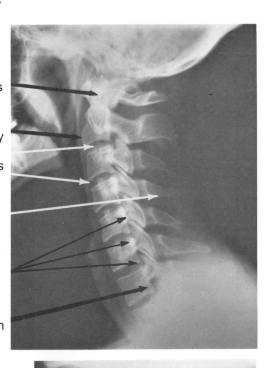

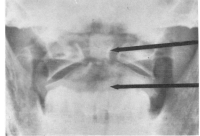

odontoid process

vertebral body

*PA view*

intervertebral (disc) spaces

spinous processes vary in
shape but are usually well
defined

alignment—check the lateral
part of the bodies

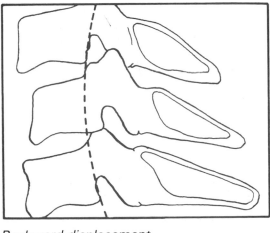

## Always check vertebral alignment

When looking at any part of the spine in the lateral view, check that
there is a smooth continuous "line" along the posterior edges of the
vertebral bodies. Check also the space between vertebrae, particularly
for narrowing.

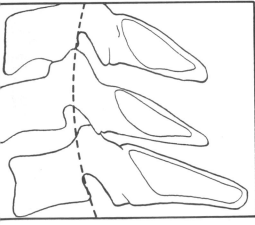

*...rward displacement*

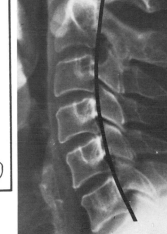

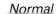

*Normal*

*Backward displacement*

148

## NORMAL THORACIC SPINE

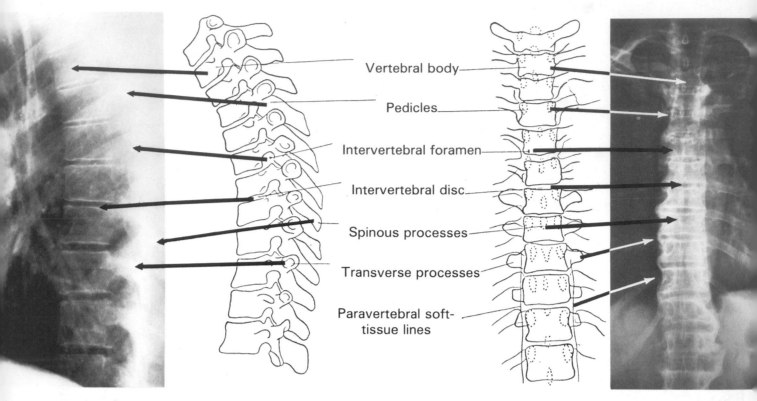

Vertebral body

Pedicles

Intervertebral foramen

Intervertebral disc

Spinous processes

Transverse processes

Paravertebral soft-
tissue lines

## NORMAL LUMBAR SPINE

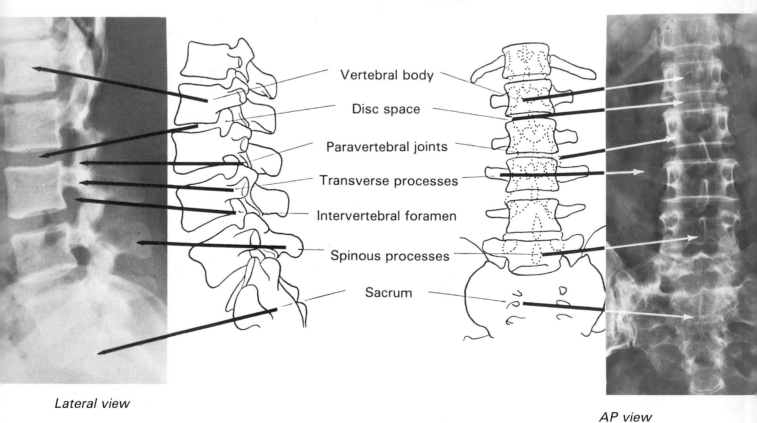

Vertebral body

Disc space

Paravertebral joints

Transverse processes

Intervertebral foramen

Spinous processes

Sacrum

*Lateral view*

*AP view*

There are normally 5 lumbar vertebrae.

There may be 4, when the 5th has become ''sacralized'', or 6, when a sacral vertebra has become ''lumbarized''.

Almost everyone has some developmental variation at the lumbosacral region (bifid spinous processes, asymmetry of the neural arch, absent or large transverse processes).

This seldom has any clinical significance unless there is vertebral displacement.

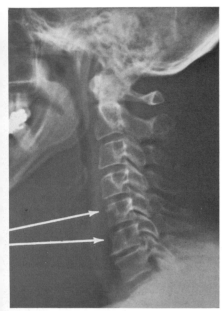

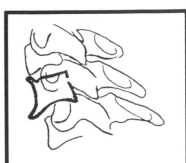

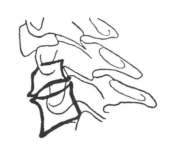

*Early*        *Late*

Many vertebrae develop bony spurs in front and also at the back as age increases. The front spurs (see arrows) are of no clinical significance. When the posterior spurs are large they can cause pressure on nerves.

Many vertebrae narrow (top to bottom) and the disc spaces narrow also. Bony spurs are always present when this happens as a result of "age" and the bones have complete outlines without any break. More than one vertebra is usually affected. This process is common and seldom causes clinical signs.

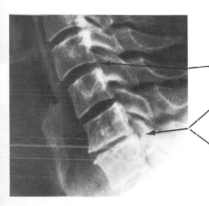

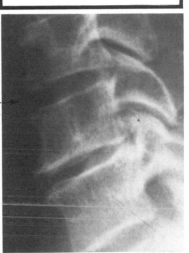

normal spaces

narrow intervertebral disc space

sclerotic (white) edges

bony spurs either side of the disc space

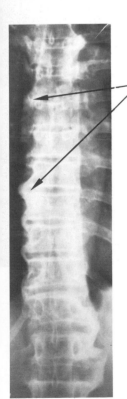

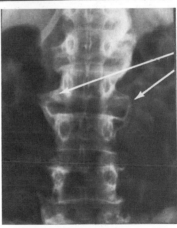

These spurs can be found on any vertebra, on the sides or front of the vertebral bodies (see arrows). They are usually asymmetrical and differ in shape. They are the result of previous injury or aging. They seldom have any clinical significance, provided the vertebral bodies are not displaced or distorted.

If so many vertebrae are involved so that the spine looks like bamboo (usually in males), this may be ankylosing spondylitis. The sacro-iliac joints will be hazy or fused, with no joint space left.

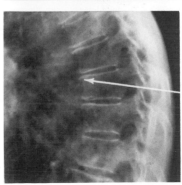

# SPINAL TRAUMA

## Different Types of Spinal Subluxation or Fracture–Dislocation

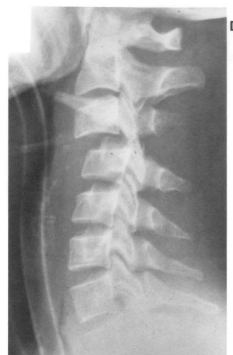

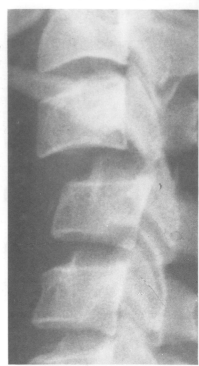

*Forward displacement of C3 on C4*

Both the anterior soft-tissue line and the posterior vertebral body curve are disrupted. This is an unstable fracture. All CERVICAL and other spinal injuries need a neurological examination.

These injuries can occur at any level in any part of the spine.

(The patient on the left has an endotracheal tube.)

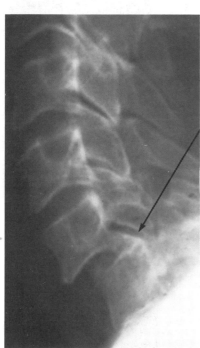

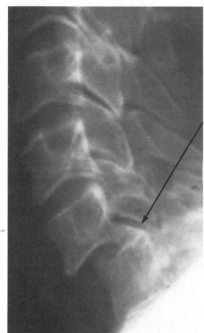

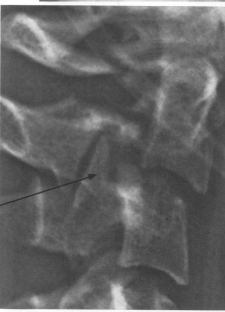

*Anterior dislocation of C6 on C7*

There must also be a fracture of the neural arch and probably spinal cord damage.

*Fracture dislocation of C2 on C3*

The neural arches have been severely fractured and the vertebral body has slipped forward.

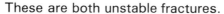

These are both unstable fractures.

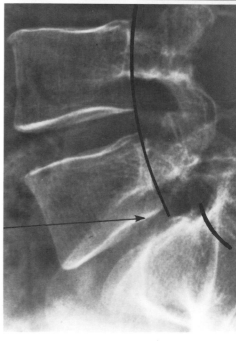

*Spondylolisthesis*

At the lumbosacral junction (and also at L4/L5) there can be a defect in the neural arch and forward subluxation of the vertebral body is possible. This may be a long-standing condition that may eventually cause backache and nerve pressure symptoms. Sometimes it is a chance finding. The forward movement on L5 can be much more pronounced than in this case, and may disturb pregnancy and stop normal delivery.

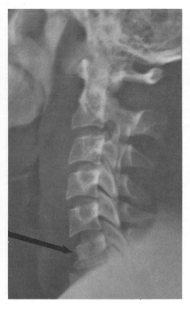

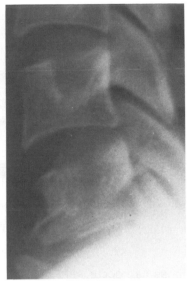

There are several different types of spinal fractures. Look carefully at the shape and alignment of each vertebral body.
One edge may be fractured. There may be no loss of disc space or vertebral displacement. This may be a relatively minor injury.

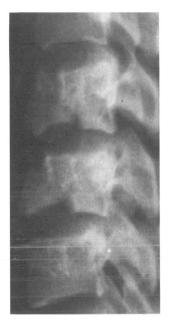

### Vertical fractures

Vertebral bodies can be fractured from top to bottom. This is always a severe injury. Note that the lowest vertebra is not correctly aligned with the one above; this means that there must be another injury, perhaps seen in the AP view.

### Wedged or compressed vertebral bodies

In the *cervical* spine this is usually a serious injury.
In the *thoracic* spine it is less serious clinically, but is painful.
In the *lumbar* spine it is usually a serious injury.
Any vertebral malalignment increases the severity of the injury at ALL levels. Every patient with a fractured vertebral body must be carefully checked neurologically and assessed clinically.

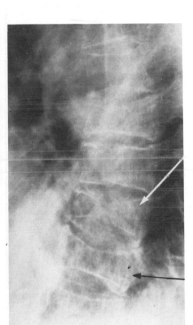

### Disc degeneration

Chronic disc narrowing. No acute injury.

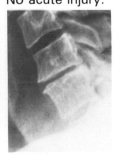

The space between the vertebral bodies (the disc space) is narrowed when the disc is damaged. This is usually *not* an acute injury and may exist for a long time without symptoms. BUT if there is a history of acute trauma, look for damage to the vertebra as well. There is a fracture of the lower part of C5 anteriorly, narrowing and flattening of the disc space, and slight posterior subluxation of C5 on C6. This was an acute injury.

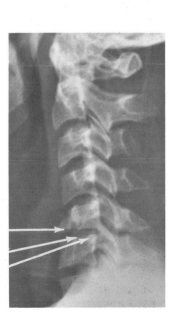

## CHANGES IN VERTEBRAL DENSITY AND OUTLINE WITHOUT INJURY

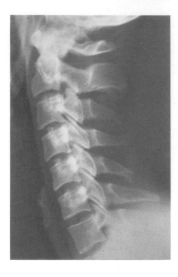

Normal vertebral bodies are smooth in outline, of the same density throughout with a white cortical line around the edge. The trabecular pattern is evenly spread through the body.

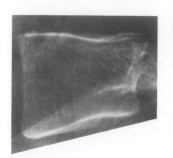

*Normal trabecular pattern*

*Destruction of vertebral body by metastasis*

When malignancy exists, the intervertebral disc space usually remains intact. As the tumour spreads, the vertebra may collapse. (You may be misled by overlying bowel gas in the lumbar region.) The disc space usually narrows when infection is present (see page 155) and there may be a paravertebral abscess.

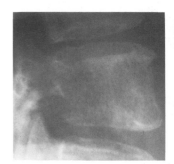

*Vertebral metastasis*

*Increased vertebral density*

Increased density of the vertebral body can be due to Paget's disease, metastasis, or infection.

The density due to metastasis is usually patchy. The vertebral body stays the same shape and the disc space remains normal. There are often multiple vertebrae involved up and down the spine (look also at films of the ribs, skull and pelvis for other metastases). Infection is seldom so widespread. In Paget's disease the vertebral body is enlarged.

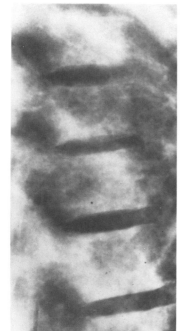

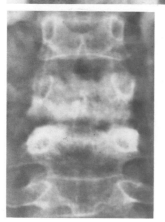

When vertebral density is due to infection usually only one or two vertebrae are involved and the vertebral outline becomes irregular. The disc space will almost always be narrowed (and irregular). There may be a paravertebral abscess (see page 154).

## Vertebral Body Outline

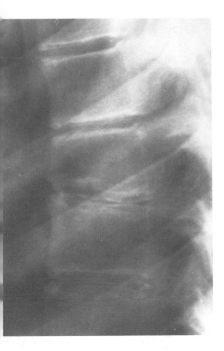

When there is irregularity of the upper or lower border of a vertebral body, with a dense white edge (most commonly in the thoracic spine) the cause is probably previous osteochondritis. This X-ray shows what is probably an old minor injury with little clinical significance. Often there are many vertebrae involved. It may be seen in the lumbar spine; it is rare in the cervical spine.

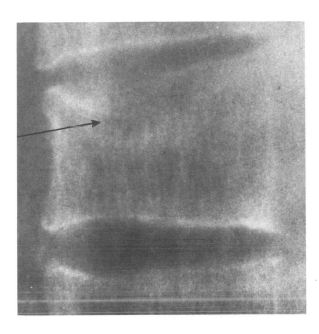

When the edge of a vertebral body is irregular but NOT dense (white) and only one vertebra is involved, this is usually due to injury or infection. If the disc space is narrowed, as in this case, infection is the most probable cause. The clinical history will help to decide.

In osteoporosis of the spine (e.g., post menopause) the width of the disc space is exaggerated and the vertebrae become biconcave.

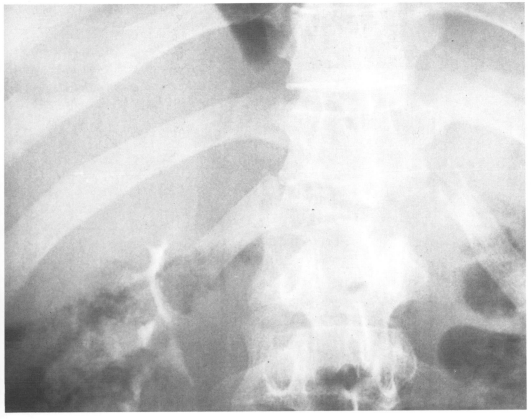

When adjoining vertebrae are destroyed, you must carefully count the ribs and pedicles. In this case the bottom left corner of the 11th vertebra is destroyed. The two 12th ribs end on a very narrow, completely crushed vertebra—the 12th. The left upper border of the 1st lumbar vertebra is also destroyed. Multiple vertebral involvement like this is usually due to infection, often tuberculous.

Did you notice that there is a large defect in the upper border of the 10th right rib? There is an abscess there too, also tuberculous.

**Paravertebral Shadows**

*Abscesses (paravertebral)*

An elliptical density on either side of the spine is almost always due to an abscess, usually tuberculous, although other infections occasionally cause similar abscesses. A very serious injury with a haematoma is an unusual cause of a density; lymphoma (e.g., Burkitt's) and neuroblastoma can also cause paravertebral densities. The densities can be unilateral or bilateral; they are often not symmetrical. As the disease progresses, it is possible to see the infected vertebra, which may be wedged, crushed, or destroyed.

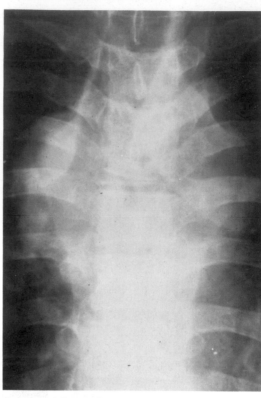

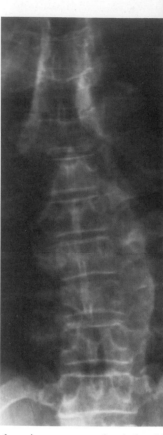

A large bilateral paravertebral abscess.

An abscess on the left side thoracic spine; no obvious lesion (yet).

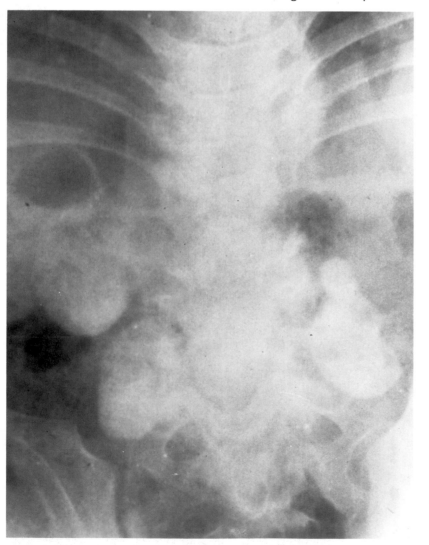

The abscess may track along the spine and eventually appear to be an inguinal or femoral hernia. The patient's clinical history will help to differentiate. Eventually the abscess will calcify and show as white paravertebral densities, usually with a granular appearance. Look carefully for the vertebral lesion. The calcification does not always mean complete healing.

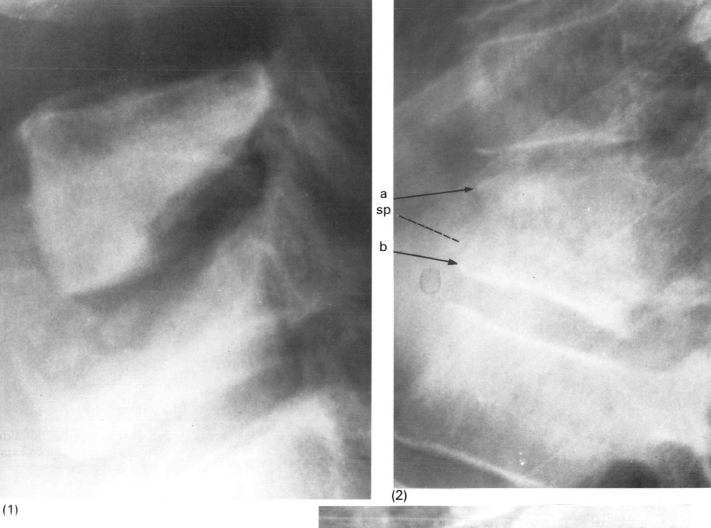

(1)

(2)

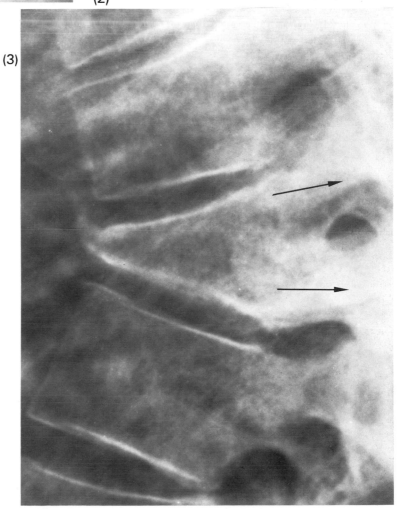

(3)

## Infection

(1) Infection of two vertebrae; the intervening disc space has almost disappeared. There are fragments of bone where the lower vertebra has collapsed centrally.

(2) As healing occurs, the two vertebrae (a and b) may fuse with loss of disc space (sp) so that they almost look like one. The solid arrows point to the upper and lower vertebrae, the interrupted line in the middle to the lost disc space.

(3) After treatment there is a solid wedge of bone made of two vertebrae. This is now well healed. You can see that there were two vertebrae because there are two neural arches (arrows) joined to the wedged (fused) bodies. Always check the neural arches in both the lateral and the AP views.

TUMOURS DO NOT AFFECT THE DISC SPACE. INFECTION USUALLY DESTROYS THE DISC SPACE.

# ABDOMINAL X-RAYS

# ABDOMINAL X-RAYS

## INDICATIONS

An abdominal radiograph is seldom of help in the diagnosis of chronic abdominal pain unless there are specific clinical indications of the etiology. A plain film is of NO assistance in confirming the diagnosis of acute ruptured ectopic pregnancy, nor will it exclude acute appendicitis, for example.

Therefore reserve radiographs for patients in whom the clinical indications strongly suggest one of the following:

(1) Obstruction of the bowel.
(2) A perforated gastric or duodenal ulcer, or perforated bowel.
(3) Renal or biliary pain, with typical colic.
(4) Foreign body, whether swallowed, following injury, or misplaced intrauterine contraceptive device.
(5) In newborn infants, failure to pass meconium, or persistent vomiting.

## QUALITY CONTROL

The supine radiograph must cover the whole of the abdomen, including the diaphragm and the pelvis. If the patient is too large for one film, use an additional film. When the clinical diagnosis is intestinal obstruction or gastrointestinal perforation, an additional erect film is necessary. Both films must include the diaphragm. The patient must be lying or standing straight. If the patient cannot stand, a cross-table decubitus film, with the patient on the left side, must be taken instead of the erect film. If perforation is suspected, add PA and lateral films of the chest.

## SEARCH PATTERN

(1) Check all the bones, particularly the lumbar spine and pelvis. Look for any change in bone density, either increased or decreased, and look for any vertebral collapse or abnormal alignment. Check the sacro-iliac joints to make sure they are clear and not hazy (fused).

(2) If there has been recent injury, look for fractures of the lower ribs and the transverse processes of the lumbar vertebrae. Make sure there is no pelvic fracture, especially either side of the pubic symphysis and around the hips.

(3) Look at the diaphragm in the erect film, for air under both sides or either side. Do not be misled by air in the stomach or colon. Confirm on the chest films, if available.

(4) Look for the psoas outlines: they cannot always be seen either on one side or on both, but this has no significance. However, the psoas lines should be straight and an asymmetrical bulge or extra line may indicate retroperitoneal haemorrhage, abscess or tumour (lymphoma).

(5) Try to identify the edge of the liver.

(6) Look for abnormal calcification, particularly in the region of the gall-bladder, pancreas, or anywhere in the urinary tract.

(7) Look at the bowel gas pattern. If distended, look at the erect film for horizontal fluid levels. Identify the anatomy; stomach first, then small bowel and colon. Make sure that there is gas in the rectum.

# MECHANICAL BOWEL OBSTRUCTION—INTESTINAL OBSTRUCTION—ILEUS

The radiographic findings must be correlated with the history and clinical examination. If the patient appears to have an acute abdomen, and yet there is difficulty in finding any specific clinical abnormality, obstruction may be considered. However, when the patient is very ill the clinical impression must dictate treatment even if the X-ray examination is not diagnostic. You cannot depend on the X-ray film to give you the diagnosis in every case. There are many causes of intestinal obstruction; only a few are illustrated.

## Normal Bowel Patterns

Try to differentiate between the small and the large bowel.

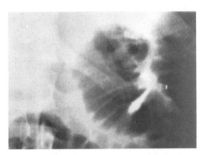

Normal (undilated) small bowel is seldom more than 3 cm wide.

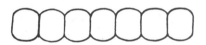

Upper small bowel

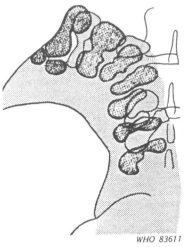

WHO 83611

The irregular pattern of gas in the colon. Compare the regular pattern of the small bowel.

The transverse colon often dips into the pelvis, even in the supine position.

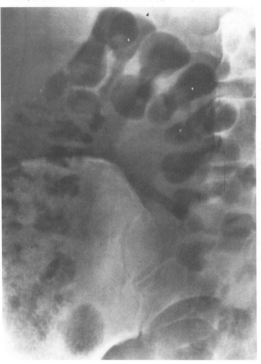

Caecum, hepatic flexure, and part of transverse colon.

Distended small bowel

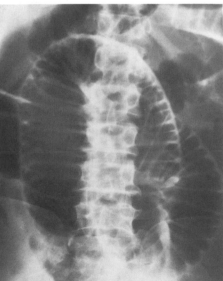

Distended colon

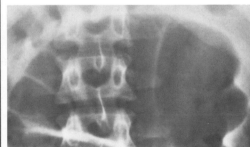

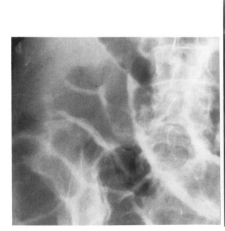

The lower ileum is smoother than the upper small bowel.

The "white lines" across the small bowel (plicae) usually divide it into equal segments.

White lines (haustra) divide the colon into very unequal segments.

## Paralytic (Adynamic) Ileus

.The bowel has ceased to function but is not mechanically obstructed.

The clinical and radiological differentiation between mechanical bowel obstruction and paralytic ileus can be VERY difficult. Careful correlation of the clinical and radiological findings is essential. Supine and erect (or decubitus) films of the abdomen are needed when paralytic ileus is suspected.

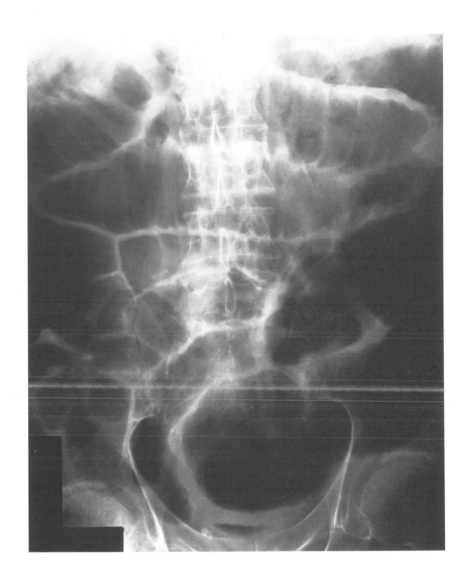

*Patient with paralytic ileus*

There is distension of both the small and the large bowel.
There is gas in the rectum and lower colon.
The stomach was distended.
(The erect film of the patient showed multiple fluid levels in the small and the large bowel.)
It is unlikely that the stomach and the rectum would both be dilated by a mechanical obstruction.

*Common causes of paralytic ileus*

Peritoneal irritation (peritonitis).
Postoperative ileus.
Postabdominal trauma.
Electrolyte disturbance
In association with severe abdominal pain, e.g., renal colic.
Diffuse peritoneal metastases.
Drugs—medicinal herbs.

---

IF THERE IS **LOCALIZED** BOWEL DISTENSION (E.G., SMALL BOWEL ONLY) OR IF THERE IS A PART OF THE BOWEL AT WHICH DISTENSION FINISHES (E.G., IN THE MID-TRANSVERSE COLON) AND IF THE RECTUM IS EMPTY WITHOUT GAS, SUSPECT **MECHANICAL** OBSTRUCTION. IF **ALL** PARTS OF THE BOWEL AND THE **STOMACH** ARE DILATED, SUSPECT **PARALYTIC ILEUS.**

# Small Bowel Obstruction

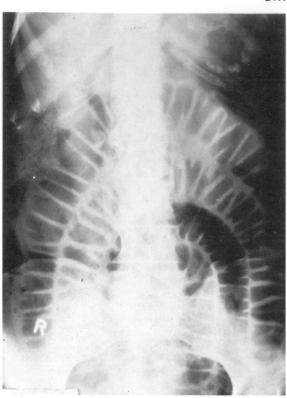

Supine

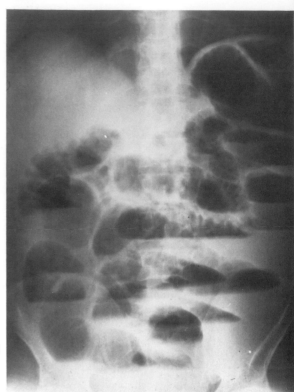

*Typical small bowel obstruction, with multiple fluid levels when erect.*

Erect

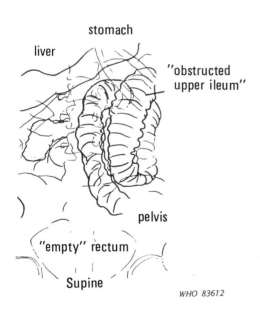

*When the ileum is obstructed the X-ray can be misleading. The lower ileum may fill with fluid and become "invisible"; the X-ray then looks like an upper small bowel obstruction, but the actual blockage can be much lower down.*

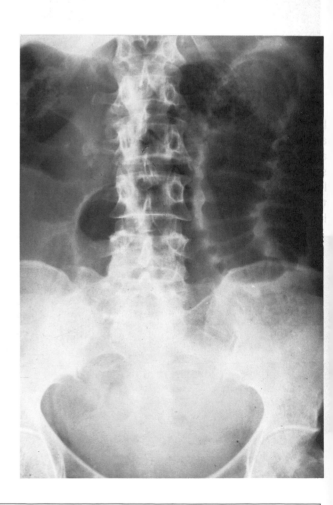

AFTER TRAUMA, A DISTENDED LOOP OF SMALL BOWEL MAY INDICATE RETROPERITONEAL OR INTRAMURAL HAEMATOMA.

## Small Bowel Obstruction *(continued)*

*Mid small bowel obstruction (supine)*

This is the typical pattern of dilated small bowel when the patient is lying supine.

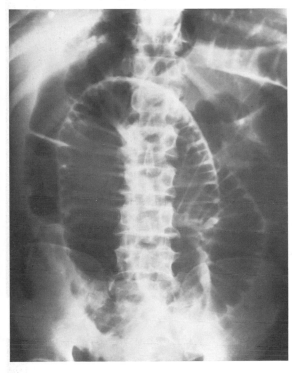

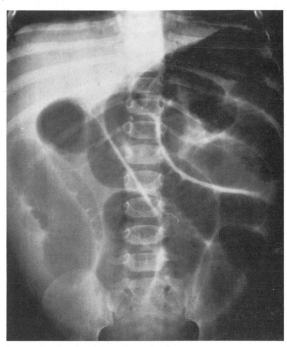

*Low small bowel obstruction (supine)*

Dilated loops of ileum which are smooth in outline (see right lower quadrant) with small loops of mid and upper ileum also (left upper quadrant). In a few hours this bowel may fill with fluid and the typical pattern may disappear (see facing page).

If the patient cannot stand, take a cross-table lateral view of the abdomen with the patient lying supine. This one shows dilated loops of small bowel with multiple fluid levels. (The umbilical hernia is coincidental.)

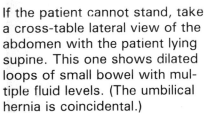

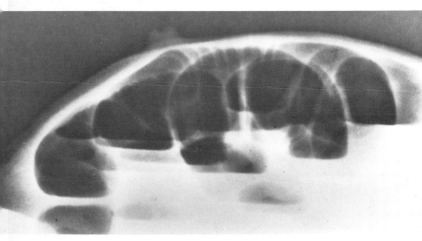

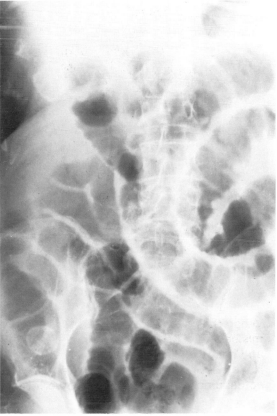

Obtruction low in the ileum due to a gallstone which has blocked the ileocaecal valve. This is known as "gallstone ileus", but is actually obstruction. There is no recognizable large bowel in this film. There may or may not be gas in the biliary tract (see page 175).

## Large Bowel Obstruction

Clinically, obstruction of the large bowel can be very insidious. The patient may notice constipation and discomfort, or occasionally diarrhoea. Later there is distension and perhaps vomiting. As the colon dilates because of obstruction, the ileum may also fill with gas.

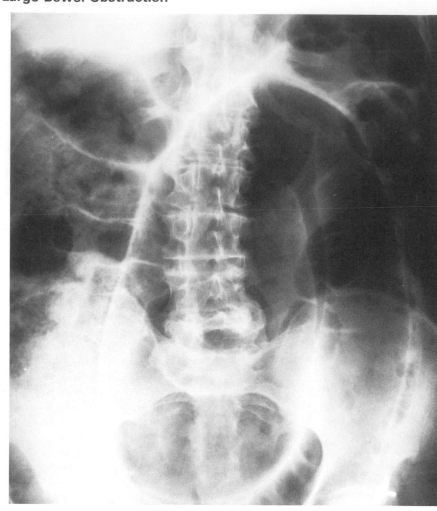

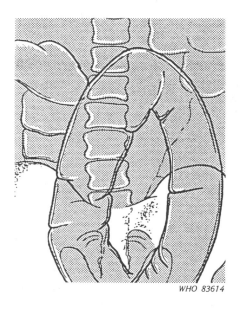

*WHO 83614*

*Volvulus of the sigmoid colon*

The large loop of distended sigmoid colon due to volvulus. The bowel is so distended it has almost lost the normal haustral pattern.

Volvulus of the sigmoid colon is a very common type of large bowel obstruction: the distended loop rises out of the pelvis, often with a visible stricture. Later the whole colon dilates.

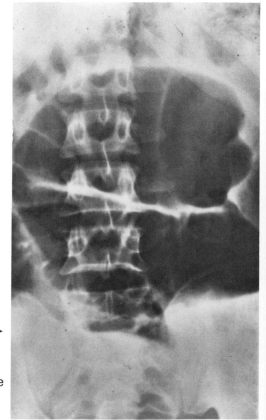

*Early sigmoid obstruction*

At this stage the transverse colon remains normal (seen here above the huge sigmoid loops). There is no gas in the pelvis below the obstruction.

## Large Bowel Obstruction *(continued)*

In this patient the bowel was obstructed in the middle of the descending colon. The splenic flexure and transverse colon are very dilated with gas and faeces. The distension has extended as far back as the caecum. The pelvis is almost empty, except for some faeces. This type of obstruction is usually due to a carcinoma of the colon or an amoeboma. However, colonic obstruction due to amoeboma or adhesions is uncommon. (Adhesions more commonly cause small bowel obstruction.)

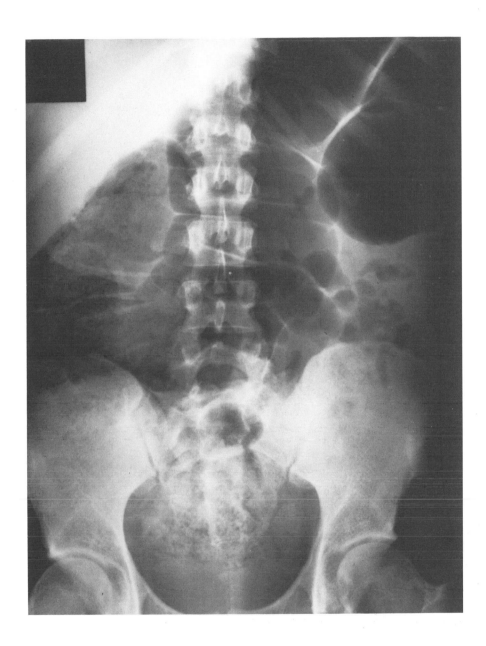

## *Megacolon*

In patients with Chagas' disease the whole colon may dilate.

In children gross dilatation may be due to aganglionosis (Hirschsprung's disease).

In any type of acute colitis (ulcerative, amoebic, tuberculous), the colon may fill with gas—a ''toxic megacolon''. The small bowel is not usually dilated. The patients are almost always extremely ill. This should be recognized, because surgery is hazardous, and contraindicated in amoebic or tuberculous colitis.

## Pseudo Obstruction (see also page 162)

Gas can normally be seen in the small bowel of children under 2 years of age, but there is no distension.
It can be very difficult to distinguish ileus and obstruction, but careful clinical and radiological investigation can usually decide. If you are not sure, but suspect ileus, re-X-ray after a few hours.

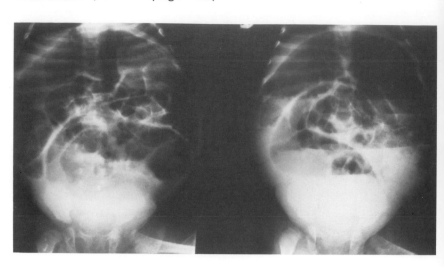

Excessive diarrhoea and vomiting in children (and occasionally in adults) can resemble obstruction. Electrolyte disturbance occurs and the bowel becomes adynamic, causing marked distension and fluid levels when erect. In children particularly, check all the hernial orifices (inguinal, femoral, umbilical) whenever a patient is vomiting continuously. Feel the abdomen for a mass, which may be felt when there is intussusception. Rehydrate and restore the child's blood chemistry before surgery. The diagnosis must be made clinically because X-rays can be very confusing.

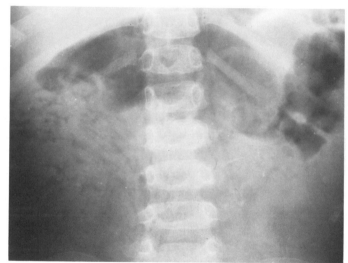

Ascaris *in the right side of the abdomen*

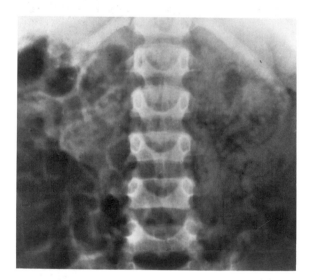

Ascaris *in the bowel (left upper quadrant)*

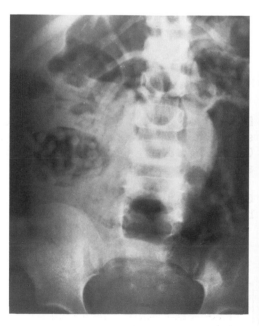

Ascaris *seen in a collection of gas (right side)*

Small bowel obstruction in children, and occasionally in adults, can be due to the roundworm, *Ascaris*. In particular, this may happen after treatment has killed the worms. On an X-ray the worms can be seen as a tangled mass with gas around them. (Do not forget that *Ascaris* may occasionally perforate the bowel wall, causing peritonitis and free air under the diaphragm.)

# PERFORATION OF THE GUT

## Free Air (Gas) in the Peritoneal Cavity (Pneumoperitoneum)

Perforation of the gastrointestinal tract is nearly always due to a peptic ulcer, occasionally to a foreign body, and rarely to trauma or to a gastric or colonic carcinoma. The bowel may perforate on account of infection, especially in typhoid (10–21 days). Diverticulitis, amoebiasis, and parasites (especially *Ascaris*) may all cause perforation. Rectal perforation is almost always due to local trauma. (Air will normally remain under the diaphragm after abdominal surgery, a stab wound or when there is an abdominal drainage tube. It can persist for two or three weeks without being significant.) When there is acute perforation there is almost always severe abdominal pain, marked tenderness to palpation and very rigid abdominal muscles.

Whenever perforation is suspected patients should be X-rayed standing or sitting. If they cannot either stand or sit, a cross-table lateral view (supine) may help, otherwise a left lateral decubitus view is necessary. These are more difficult to evaluate. In the erect view (only) look for gas under the diaphragm, showing as a thin or thick black line.

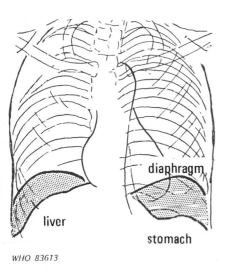

WHO 83613

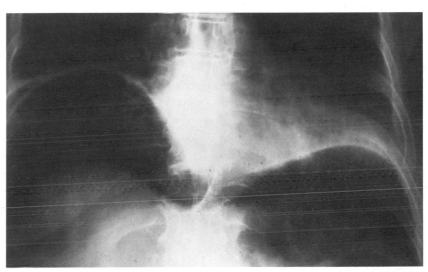

*Erect chest X-ray*

Large amount of subphrenic gas from a perforated gastric ulcer.

Differentiate: on the left side, gas in the stomach. There is usually a fluid level also. On the right side, the colon can occasionally slip above the liver. Look for the haustra.

Gas from perforation is usually bilateral, but may be asymmetrical.

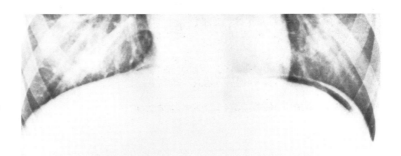

Much less subphrenic gas from a small perforation: remember the patient must be ERECT before this can be recognized.

**PERFORATION?**
TAKE **ERECT** FILM WHENEVER POSSIBLE.
(HORIZONTAL BEAM.)

## FOREIGN BODIES

Apart from intrauterine contraceptive devices (IUDs), most foreign bodies are swallowed or, occasionally, follow trauma. All metals and some plastics are radiopaque. (Do not forget tablets and capsules: see facing page.)

Any opaque object in the patient's pocket or on the skin may show on the X-ray and appear to be within the abdomen. If there is any doubt, take off all the patient's clothing and cover with a sheet or blanket. If the foreign body is in the muscles, a lateral view will decide whether it is in the abdominal muscles anteriorly or in the back or buttocks.

Metal foreign bodies which have been swallowed are nearly always easily seen, even when in front of the spine. If you are sure that the patient has swallowed a foreign body which should be opaque and yet you cannot see it on the supine film, repeat the film with the patient prone or slightly oblique. Make quite sure that he does not breathe during the exposure. If nothing is visible within the abdomen, take a lateral film of the neck, and if it is still not seen, take PA and lateral films of the chest.

Most foreign bodies pass readily through the alimentary tract and reach the rectum without causing clinical signs. X-rays, particularly repeat X-rays, are seldom needed unless the patient develops severe abdominal pain.

Intrauterine contraceptive devices all have radiopaque markers. There are many different patterns: they can escape from the uterus and may be found in the pelvis or anywhere in the abdomen. They seldom cause symptoms even in the peritoneal cavity. The exact location in the pelvis can be difficult to decide in some cases.

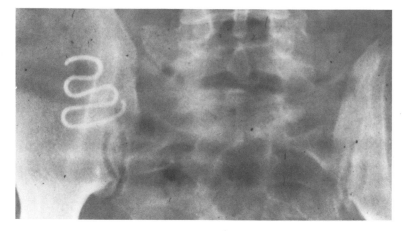 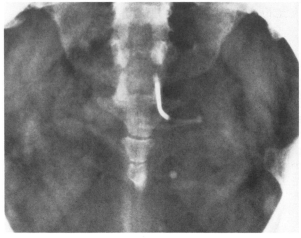

*Two different designs of IUD in the pelvis*
The spiral loop on the left is probably outside the uterine cavity.

IF YOU HAVE ANY DOUBT ABOUT A FOREIGN BODY, RE-X-RAY THE PATIENT WITHOUT CLOTHING OR COVERING, OR, ALTERNATIVELY, TAKE A LATERAL VIEW TO MAKE SURE THAT THE FOREIGN BODY IS ACTUALLY INSIDE THE PATIENT.

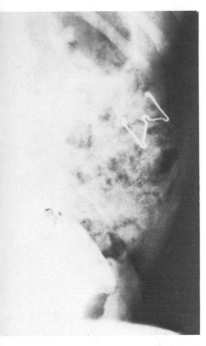

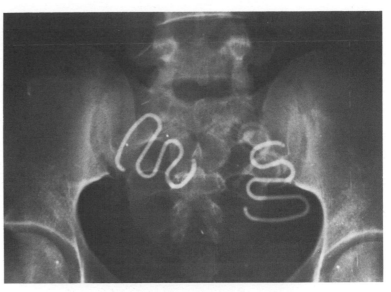

This IUD migrated to the splenic region.

This patient's doctor did not use X-rays to check when the patient said she had "lost her IUD". He put in a second one! Both are outside the uterus in the peritoneal cavity and therefore useless as contraceptives.

Remember that many TABLETS and CAPSULES are radiopaque, and after they have been swallowed may be seen anywhere in the alimentary tract and therefore anywhere in the abdomen. They can usually be recognized by their round or capsular shape. Medical powders—e.g., antacids—may also be seen scattered through the bowel as fine granules or in clumps. Oral cholecystography tablets may not be absorbed and may become scattered as granules throughout the bowel. The clinical history will help in all cases.

## ABDOMINAL CALCIFICATIONS

There are many different causes of calcification within the abdomen, and many types of calcification have a characteristic shape and/or position. The clinical history is sometimes important because gallstones and renal stones often have caused pain in the past or are currently causing it, whereas most other calcifications are entirely painless and their existence is unknown to the patient.

### Search Pattern and Differential Diagnosis

The position of the calcification is very important:

(a) *Upper abdomen:* costal cartilages, gallstones, renal stones, nephrocalcinosis, phleboliths in the kidney, renal tumours, pancreatic calcification, vascular calcification, hydatid cysts or granulomas in the liver or spleen, lymph nodes.

(b) *Mid-abdomen:* ureteric stones, low-lying gallstones, vascular calcification (particularly aortic), hydatid cysts or other parasitic conditions (porocephalosis, guinea-worm infestation), mesenteric lymph nodes.

(c) *Pelvic area:* fibroids, lymph nodes, ureteric or bladder calculi, buttock injections, dermoids, vascular calcifications, including phleboliths.

## Upper Abdomen

*Right side*

Gallstones: often laminated, multi-angular, may be single or multiple.
Liver: hydatid cysts, calcified granulomas.
Costal cartilages: usually peripheral, often linear.
Adrenals: close to spine (LI—L2) above the kidney.

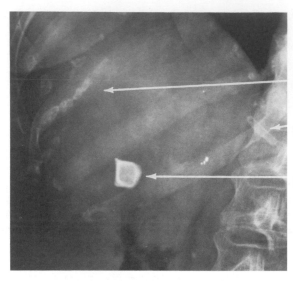

(1) costal cartilages

(2) end of nasogastric tube

(3) single laminated faceted gallstone

*Kidney stones* (see also page 190)

These must always lie over the renal shadow whatever the position of the patient. They can be:
(1) large, "staghorn" and shaped like renal pelvis and calyces;
(2) small, like one calyx;
(3) solitary, round, smooth or rough.

Do not forget that a gallstone may lie over the right kidney; take a lateral view to differentiate if necessary.

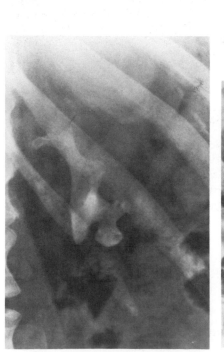
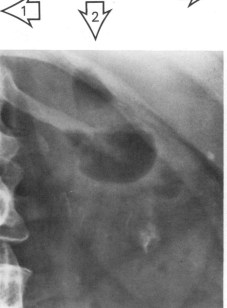
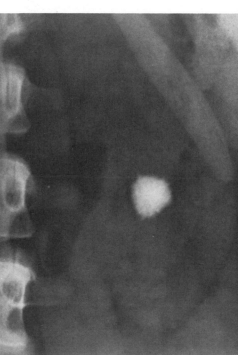

**Upper Abdomen** *(continued)*

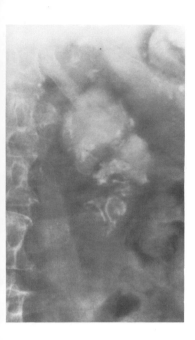

*Irregular calcification*

Irregular amorphous calcification with distorted renal outline due to a tuberculous (or other) infection. The kidney is shrunken.

Linear and curled calcification can also occur in renal malignancies, especially in children. The kidney is then enlarged, not shrunken as in infection.

*Hydatid cysts*

These can be in the spleen, kidney, liver (either right or left lobe) or anywhere in the peritoneum. They can be any size, but usually calcify like an egg, and may be crushed. Other types of renal, splenic, or hepatic cysts seldom calcify.

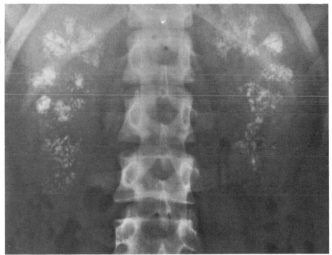

*Bilateral radiating ''brush'' calcification in the renal ducts and papillae, due to medullary sponge kidney*

Other causes of parenchymal calcification (e.g., tuberculosis, metabolic disorder, cortical necrosis) are more amorphous.

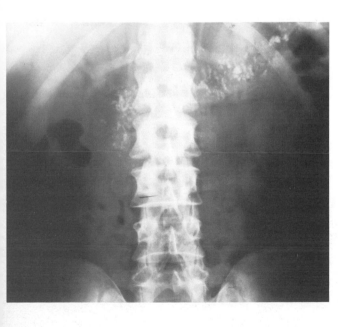

*Pancreatic calcification*

Calcification across the upper abdomen is usually in the pancreas and follows pancreatic anatomy. It can be due to childhood malnutrition or result from chronic pancreatitis, often due to chronic intake of excess alcohol.

Scattered multiple calcifications across the abdomen are usually due to parasites, either *Porocephalus (Armillifer armillatus)* or the linear or convoluted calcification of guinea-worm (see next page).

## Lower Abdomen

The commonest types are ureteric calculi, lymph nodes, bladder calculi, and phleboliths.

*Lymph node calcification (thin white arrows)*

This can be confusing (see page 191).

*Ureteric calculi*

These must lie within the anatomical line of the ureters (see page 191).

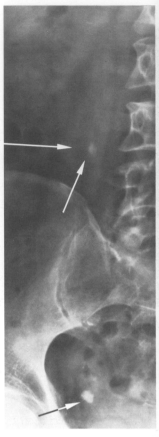

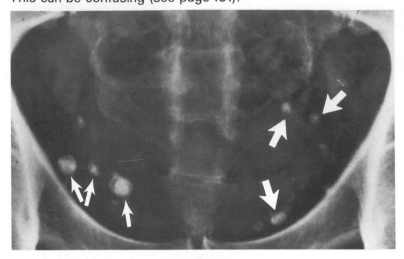

*Phleboliths (broad white arrows)*

These are round, usually like a ring with a "hollow" or less dense centre. They are usually multiple, of different sizes and densities and not all within the line of the ureters (see page 191).

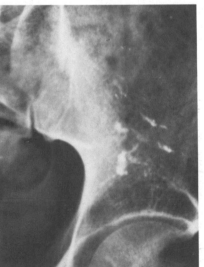

*Injection granulomas*

Injections into the buttocks calcify into "cysts" or linear shadows. These are usually bilateral but not symmetrical.

*Calcified guinea-worms*

These may be seen in the buttocks (or any other muscle). They are usually coiled "strings of beads". At this stage the parasites are dead, but there may be others in the body that are still viable following a recent infection.

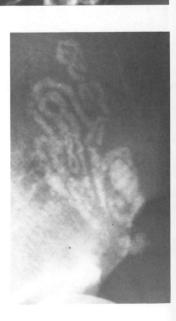

**Pelvis**

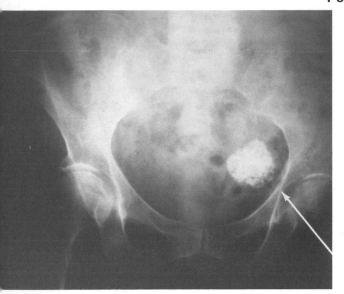

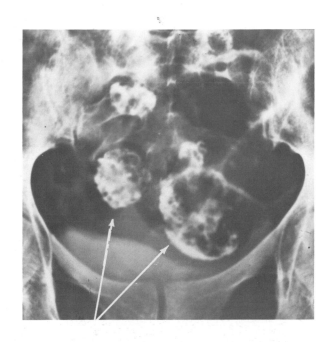

*Uterine fibroids*

Uterine fibromyomata (fibroids) may be single or multiple, small or large.

*Dermoid cysts*

These are usually in the pelvis, but can be elsewhere in the abdomen. Most dermoids have a "tooth" or "bone" with translucent fat around them. The dermoid will usually be larger than it seems radiologically.

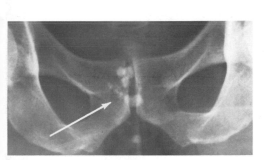

*Calculi in the prostate*

There may be calculi in the prostate, behind or below the pubic symphysis. They are of no clinical significance and do not indicate prostatic infection or enlargement.

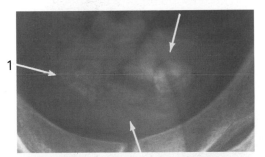

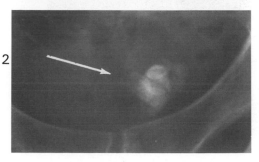

*Bladder calculi (1 and 2)*

These can be single or multiple. They may change position as the patient moves (see also page 192).

# GALL-BLADDER

If gall-bladder disease is suspected, first take a film of the abdomen. Look particularly at the right side of the abdomen for calcified stones or gas in the biliary tract.

## Gallstones (calculi)

These are either round or faceted. They can be multi-layered. If the film is taken with the patient erect, the gallstones may be even lower than the right iliac crest.

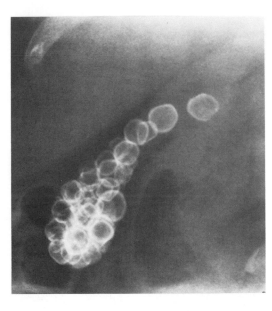

Faceted stones within the gall-bladder

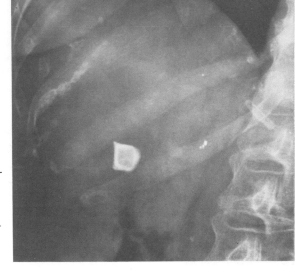

Isolated gall-stone

(Note costal cartilage calcification above it.)

## Differential diagnosis

Other calcifications may be confused with gallstones (see pages 170–171).

(A) Pancreatic calcification usually crosses the lumbar spine to the left and is usually multiple.

(B) Mesenteric lymph nodes can occur anywhere in the abdomen, but are often on the right side, low down.

(C) Renal stones can be differentiated by a lateral view because the gall-bladder is anteriorly and the kidneys are posteriorly alongside the lumbar spine.

Calcified costal cartilages are usually bilateral and extended beyond and above the gall-bladder area. They do not alter position when the patient is erect.

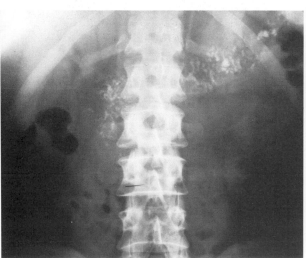

(A) Pancreatic calcification

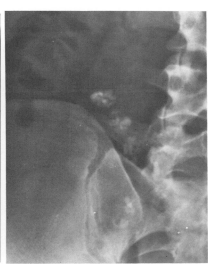

(B) Calcified lymph nodes

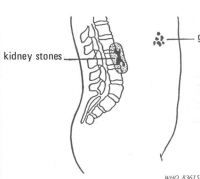

WHO 83615

(C) Gallstones lie anteriorly in lateral view

## Gas in the Biliary Tract

This is only of significance in acutely ill patients, when it is almost always due to infection. If the patient is not ill, gas may be seen after gastrointestinal surgery or the development of a fistula between the gall-bladder and the duodenum.

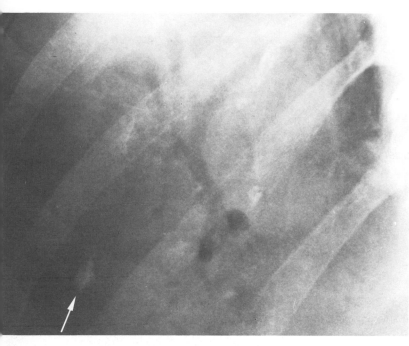

It is recognized by the branching pattern seen against the liver. (The calcification seen laterally in this film is in the costal cartilage at the end of a rib.)

costal calcification

### Hydatid cyst

Calcification in the liver outside the gall-bladder may be due to a hydatid cyst. If the calcification is more medial or lower down, exclude renal calcification (see pages 189-190).

cyst

gall-bladder

Calcification can be seen in the wall of the gall-bladder after infection: it will always be in the shape of all or part of the gall-bladder. Occasionally bile in the gall-bladder is radiopaque, as in a cholecystogram. This is probably of little clinical significance. Gallstones are usually in the gall-bladder and conform to that shape (see illustration opposite). Sometimes they are in the cystic or common bile ducts. Then the patients will nearly always have pain (colic) and may be jaundiced.

## Cholecystograms: the Gall-Bladder with Contrast

Contrast studies can help to demonstrate gall-bladder disease, particularly gallstones which cannot be seen on routine films because they do not contain enough calcium. NEVER do this investigation in jaundiced patients. Remember that in some parts of the world, children may be jaundiced because there are *Ascaris* in the common bile duct.

*Preparation*

The patient should swallow the cholecystography tablets (usually iopanoic acid or equivalent) in the dose directed on the package. These should be swallowed with water in the evening, *12 hours* before the examination. After this the patient should take NO food and drink *only water* until after the X-ray films have been taken the next morning.

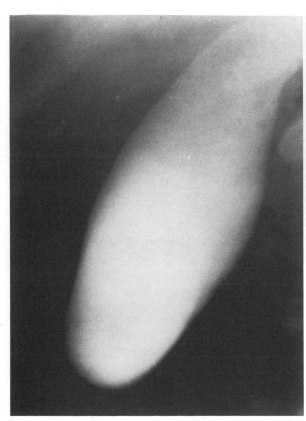

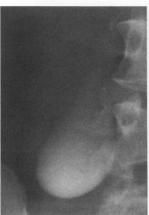

*Normal gall-bladder low in the abdomen*

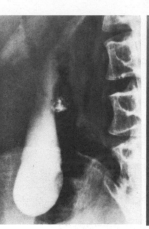

When the gall-bladder contracts, the cystic and common bile ducts may be seen.
However, failure to show the ducts does not mean disease.

*Normal gall-bladder*

If there is bowel gas overlying the gall-bladder, stand the patient erect or take a decubitus film with the patient lying on the right side (see facing page).

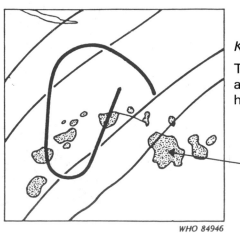

*Kinked gall-bladder*

The gall-bladder can appear kinked, but this has no clinical significance.

gas bubbles

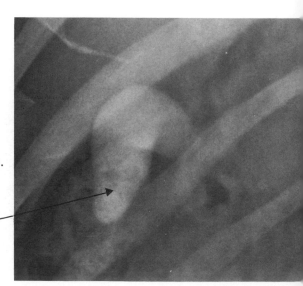

WHO 84946

## Cholecystograms: the Gall-Bladder with Contrast *(continued)*

*Gall-bladder not seen 12 hours after the tablets have been taken*

If the gall-bladder cannot be seen on films taken 12 hours after the patient has taken tablets, there are several possible explanations: (1) ask the patient whether the tablets have been swallowed; (2) ask if the patient has had diarrhoea or vomiting, as this may impair absorption of the tablets.

If you cannot see the gall-bladder in the morning after the tablets have been taken, give the patient a second dose of tablets the same evening (unless the first dose has caused significant upset). Re-X-ray 12 hours after the second dose of tablets. If the gall-bladder still cannot be seen, it is probably diseased.

(A)

(B)

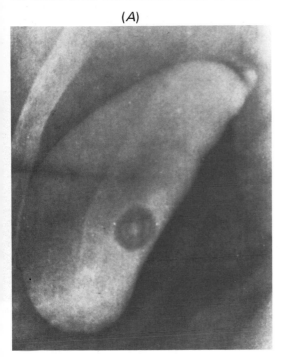

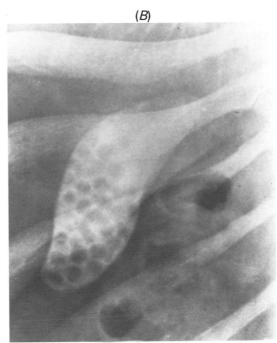

(A) Solitary gallstone.
(B) Multiple faceted stone.
(C) Layered stones in an erect view.
(D) Erect view; there is bowel gas over the lower part of the gall-bladder.
(E) Decubitus view of the same patient lying on the right side; two stones are quite clearly shown, and the gas has moved above the gall-bladder.

(C)                    (D)                    (E)

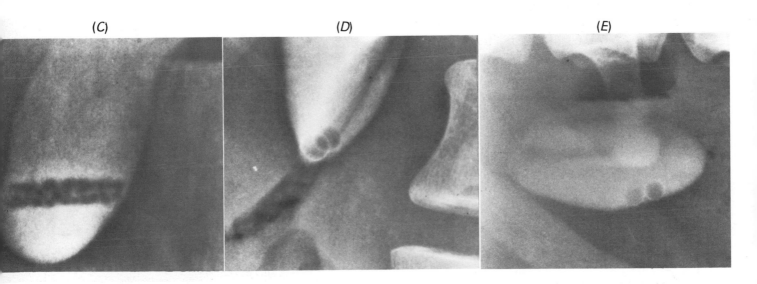

# OBSTETRIC X-RAYS

# OBSTETRIC X-RAYS

## INDICATIONS

---

A RADIOGRAPH OF THE PELVIS SHOULD **NEVER** BE TAKEN TO DIAGNOSE EARLY PREGNANCY.

---

Because of the potential hazards of radiation damage to the growing fetus, the only indications for X-ray examination occur in the last weeks of pregnancy. *X-rays should only be taken when the information will affect management.* Unlike ultrasound studies, which have no known danger, *there can be NO routine use of X-rays in obstetrics.*

In particular, in cases of antepartum haemorrhage, placental localization by radiography is difficult and is NOT recommended.

Is there any possibility that the delivery will not be normal?
Does the patient need to go to a special centre for delivery?

Radiology will help you to answer the following clinical questions:

(1) *Malposition* can be confirmed or identified.

(2) *Multiple pregnancy* can be recognized in patients who are difficult to palpate.

(3) *Fetal abnormalities* or malpositions which are significant obstetrically can be recognized.

(4) *Disproportion* can be confirmed in the last four weeks of pregnancy.
Radiography for disproportion is rarely necessary or useful except in the following patients:

   (a) those who have a history of previous obstructed labour;
   (b) those who may be too small on clinical examination (if the pelvis is DEFINITELY small by clinical measurement, there is NO reason for a subsequent X-ray examination);
   (c) those who are known to have had a pelvic fracture.

(5) *Trial labour.* There may be a need for X-ray examination in trial labour when:

   (a) the pelvic size is possibly too small;
   (b) a breech or other abnormal presentation is suspected;
   (c) there is suspected fetal abnormality, especially hydrocephalus.

## INDICATIONS *(continued)*

(6) *Fetal maturation.* It is possible to assess the age of the fetus, but this can be difficult and films must be of excellent quality (see page 186).

(*a*) If the lower femoral epiphysis is visible, the fetus is about 36 weeks or more.
(*b*) When the upper tibial epiphysis is visible, the fetus is mature (at full term).

Remember that there is considerable biological variation and these estimates are only very approximate. You must also use your clinical judgement, ascertain the date of the last menstrual period, assess the size of the uterus clinically, etc.

(7) *Fetal death.* It is not easy to recognize fetal death from an X-ray film. When the fetus dies the skull collapses and there is overlap of the skull bones radiologically. BUT similar overlap also occurs normally as soon as labour commences.

## CHOICE OF RADIOGRAPHIC PROJECTION

FOR ALL OBSTETRIC X-RAYS THE PATIENT MUST HAVE AN EMPTY BLADDER.

(1) *For fetal presentation or multiple pregnancy.* A prone abdomen, if possible. If this is too difficult, it should be taken supine.
(2) *Is there disproportion?* There are several methods of obtaining the exact pelvic size but these are complicated. Significant disproportion can be easily judged on an erect lateral projection after 36 weeks. The mother's lumbosacral angle and pubic symphysis must be visible, with the fetal head for comparison (see page 185).
(3) *For fetal age or abnormality.* Prone oblique position.

## QUALITY CONTROL

NEVER REPEAT THE FILM UNLESS ABSOLUTELY ESSENTIAL.

In all films it should be possible to see the wall of the uterus and the fetal bones. (If the fetus is moving there will be blurring.)

The prone oblique view decreases movement and is more likely to show the fetal knees clearly. However, this projection is of no value for assessing disproportion and is not helpful for showing the presentation or a multiple pregnancy.

## SEARCH PATTERN

Look at the maternal pelvis and spine for deformity.
Find the fetal spine and head.
What is the lie (presentation) of the fetus?
Is there more than one fetus?
Is the neck extended or flexed?
If in the breech position, are the legs extended or flexed? (Both or one?)
Look for the fetal knees and the epiphyses at the lower end of the femur/upper end of the tibia.

## FETAL PRESENTATIONS—ABNORMALITIES—MULTIPLE PREGNANCIES

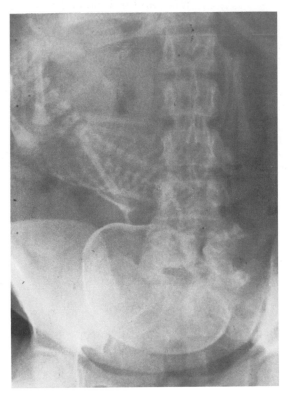

*Vertex, extended neck*

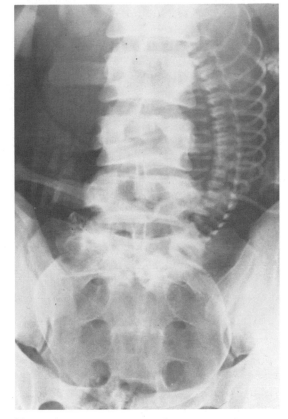

*Normal vertex presentation*

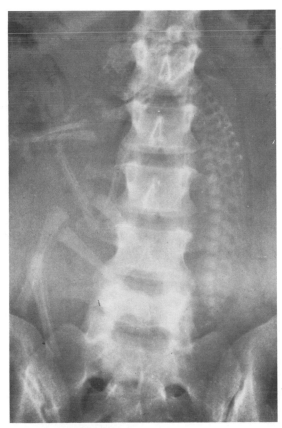

*Anencephalic fetus*

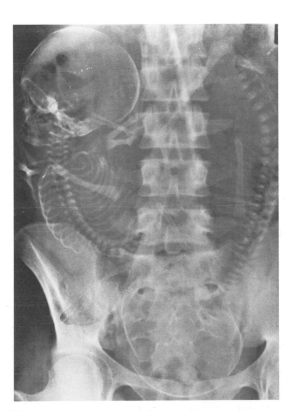

*Twins*

## FETAL PRESENTATIONS—ABNORMALITIES—MULTIPLE PREGNANCIES *(continued)*

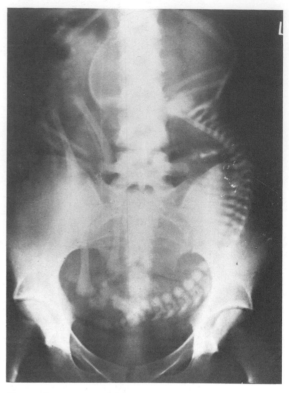

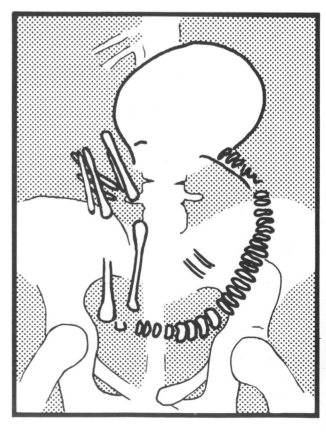

*Transverse lie*

*Breech presentation*

Beware of considering the head hydrocephalic in breech presentation if the view is taken supine. The fetal head is geometrically enlarged as it is a long way from the film. This fetus has both legs extended, which will prevent delivery unless corrected.

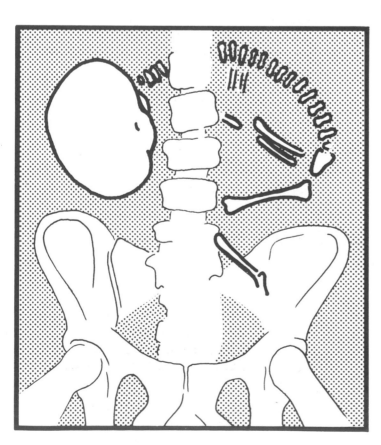

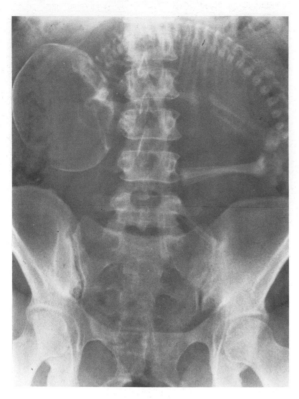

## DISPROPORTION

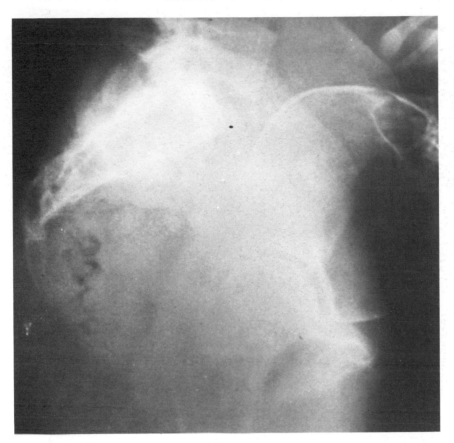

To find out whether the fetal head will pass through the pelvis, an erect lateral view is helpful in the last 3–4 weeks of pregnancy with a vertex presentation. Direct comparison can be made between the diameter of the fetal skull and the maternal pelvic inlet (promontory to pubis). If the fetus is clearly too large, normal delivery is unlikely. This is not useful with breech or other abnormalities.

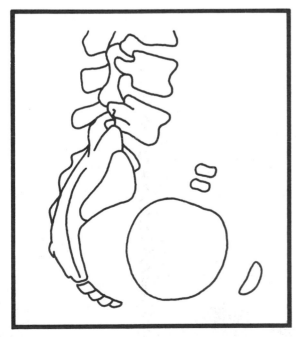

*Lateral pelvis*

Head engaged. No disproportion.

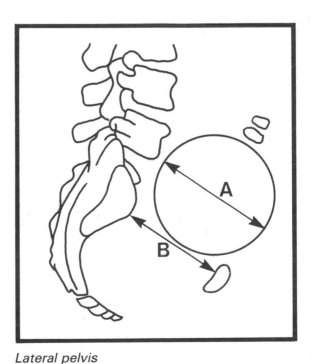

*Lateral pelvis*

Head high. Transverse A greater than inlet transverse B. Disproportion.

## APPEARANCE OF FETAL MATURATION

### Ossific Centres

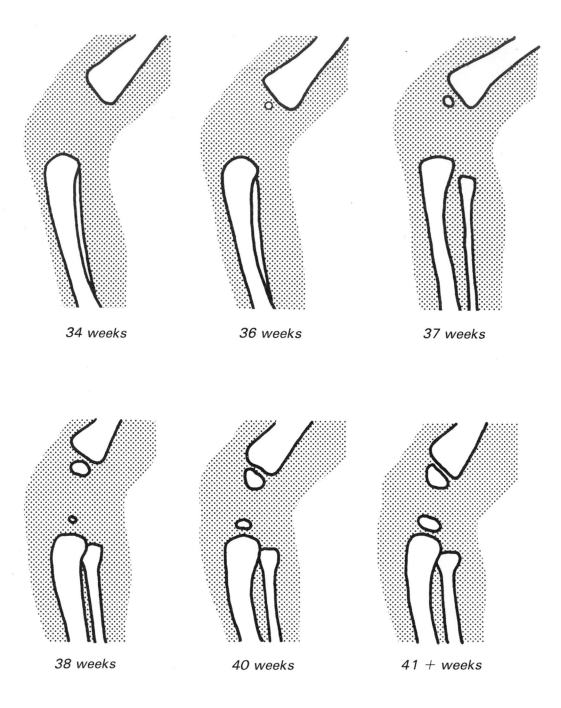

34 weeks          36 weeks          37 weeks

38 weeks          40 weeks          41 + weeks

These maturation dates are approximate.

**URINARY TRACT—KIDNEYS, URETERS, BLADDER, URETHRA**

# URINARY TRACT—KIDNEYS, URETERS, BLADDER, URETHRA

## PLAIN FILM

### Quality Control

The first film is always of the abdomen without contrast. It must show the 11th rib and the pubic symphysis. If the patient is too large, add another film of the pelvis.

### Search Pattern

Look first at all the bones, the ribs, spine, and pelvis, to exclude infection, metastases, or other abnormality. Then look at the psoas contour. It is not always visible, which is not important, but a change in the normal straight line of the psoas muscle is usually significant. Identify the kidney size and shape, then the bladder. Note any calcifications.

*Excess faeces obscuring detail*

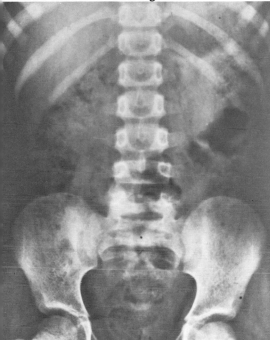

If the colon contains, too much faeces or gas, the kidneys may be obscured and calculi in the ureter or bladder may be missed. Empty the bowel and re-X-ray.

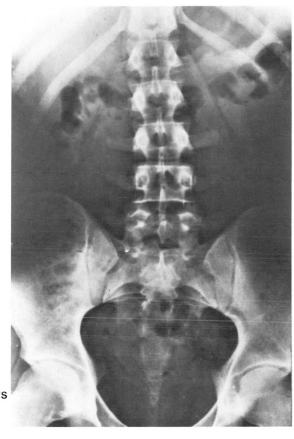

*Normal abdomen*

Skeleton, left psoas muscle, and kidneys are clearly visible.

The kidneys should be the same size (the left is usually higher than the right) and smooth in outline. There is usually a smooth bulge on the lateral side of the left kidney. Any other local outward bulge suggests a renal cyst or tumour. Any shrinkage, local or of the whole kidney, suggests chronic infection.

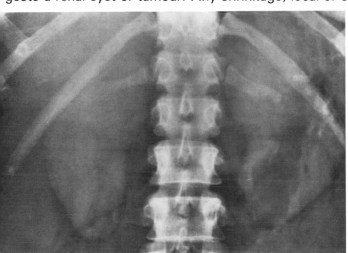

*Normal, smooth symmetrical kidneys*

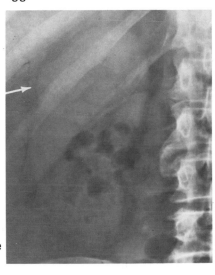

*Localized kidney bulge*
A localized bulge due to a renal cyst or tumour. (For a shrunken kidney, see page 200.)

## Calcification in the Renal Area

Renal calculi will always lie over the renal outline what-ever the position of the patient. Oblique or lateral films will help to differentiate renal stones from gallstones or other calcification.

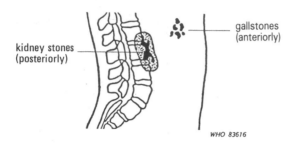

Kidney stones can be single or multiple, smooth or rough. They are usually quite dense and can be bilateral. They may be in the shape of the renal calyx or pelvis. When large they are called "staghorn" calculi; these cause repeated urinary infections. Small fragments may break off into the ureter and cause renal colic or obstruction.

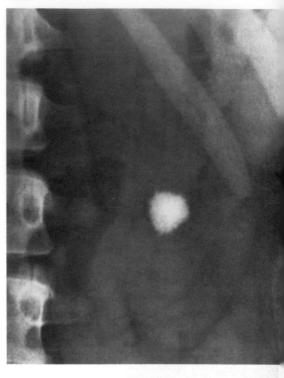

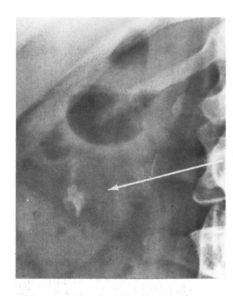

*Small calyceal calculus*

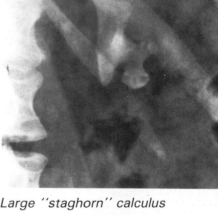

*Large "staghorn" calculus*

The kidney will be damaged by repeated infection.

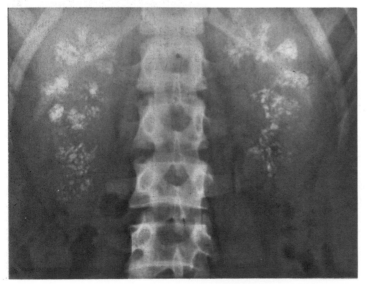

This type of calcification is not in the renal pelvis or calyces. It is due to medullary sponge kidney; it is often bilateral, but not always symmetrical. It is always within the renal contours and does not need treatment unless there are also calculi.

# Ureters

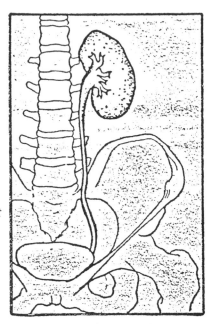

*The normal position of the urinary tract*
Calculi may be seen anywhere.

## Search pattern

Look along the line of the ureters, which lie over the lumbar transverse processes on either side of the spine and then curve outward slightly before entering the bladder. Calculi may be anywhere along this tract.

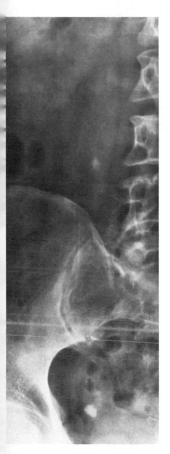

## Ureteric calculi

These can be single or multiple. In this patient, there is one in the mid-ureter and one just above the bladder. Ureteric calculi may be very small and may not be visible radiographically. They are easily obscured by heavy bowel shadow. If there is good clinical indication, a contrast examination may be necessary.

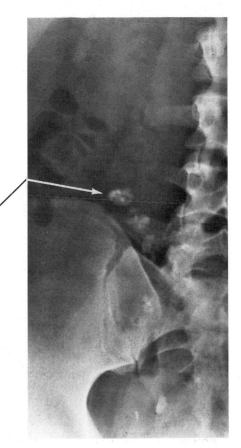

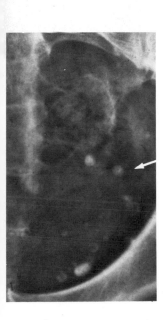

## Differential diagnosis

Ureteric calculi must be distinguished from lymph nodes and phleboliths. Lymph node calcification can be single or multiple, but is seldom all in the line of the ureter.
Phleboliths are almost always multiple ring shadows of different densities and sizes, and the majority are within the pelvis. Sometimes a contrast examination is needed to differentiate phleboliths from calculi.

## Pelvis

*The bladder*

This can often be recognized as a "ball" within the pelvis, even without contrast. Empty before a contrast study.

*Bladder calculi*

These can be single or multiple, large or small. They are often laminated. (See also page 205.)

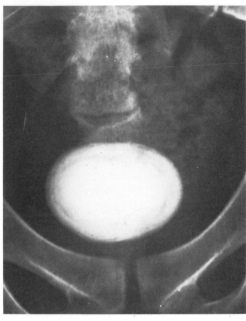

A single laminated bladder stone. This patient is likely to have chronic cystitis.

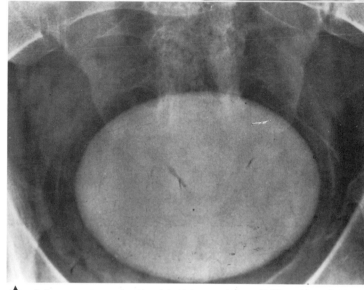

A large stone in the bladder, with calcification due to schistosomiasis.

Bladder calcification is almost always due to schistosomiasis (see also pages 205–206).

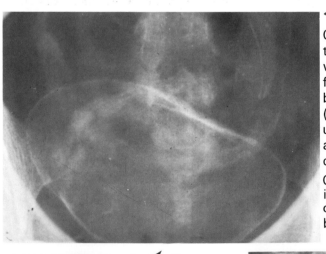

Calcification in the wall of a full bladder (both ureters are also calcified).

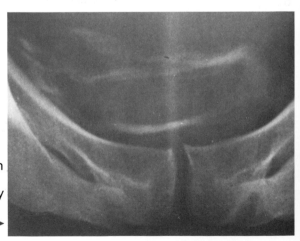

Calcification in the wall of an empty bladder.

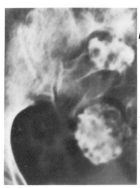

*Fibroids*

*Dermoids*

These can be recognized (see page 173).

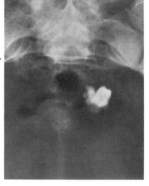

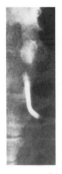

*Intrauterine contraceptive devices* (see pages 168–169).

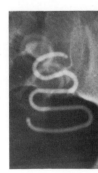

# UROGRAPHY: CONTRAST EXAMINATION OF THE KIDNEYS, URETERS, AND BLADDER

## Major Clinical Indications

Haematuria.
Loin pain (unexplained).
Renal colic.
Recurrent urinary infection.
Suspected renal mass.
Ill-defined abdominal pain is NOT an indication for urography.

## Preparation

For acute (emergency) cases no preparation is needed.
For others, give a strong laxative for two evenings before; this will help to clean the bowel and reduce the amount of gas. Make sure that the patient drinks plenty of fluid.

## Technical Procedure

First take a plain film of the whole abdomen. Check for quality and look for any significant calcification or other abnormality. If there has been recent trauma, exclude fractures of the lower ribs, lumbar transverse process, or pelvis. If there is calcification partially obscured by gas in the bowel, take further views (see pages 170–171).

After the plain films have been examined, and if the diagnosis is not obvious, the contrast medium can be injected intravenously. This decision is the doctor's responsibility.

Urographic contrast medium may occasionally cause reactions. Ask the patient if he has ever had this examination previously and if there was any reaction. Most reactions are mild, a feeling of heat and a strange taste in the mouth. Sometimes there is mild urticaria, itching, and nausea. Usually this does not require treatment; if the reaction is severe treat according to instructions on pages 15–16. (SEE YELLOW PAGES AT THE BEGINNING OF THIS BOOK.)

If the reaction is serious, which is rare, the patient may suffer from vascular collapse, respiratory distress, laryngeal oedema, or even cardiac arrest. Use cardiopulmonary resuscitation (see yellow pages 19–23) and follow the instructions for such emergencies. (Death can occur with intravenous contrast injections in about 1:30 000 injections.)

Many intravenous urographic contrast solutions are available and they vary in concentration. Check the description and the dose on the packet. Avoid solutions which are primarily made for angiography (they are too strong) or cystography (they are too weak).

The normal adult dose is between 40 ml and 100 ml. For children aged between 2 and 15 years, the dose is up to 1 ml per kg of body-weight.

## Technical Procedure *(continued)*

Inject the full dose rapidly; it MUST be given intravenously. There will be much local pain if it is given outside the vein.

Take the first film as soon as the injection is finished—this must be within 3 minutes of starting.

Look at the film to see the kidneys.

Take the next film 10 minutes after the injection started. Look at the kidneys, ureters, and bladder. If they can all be clearly seen, no more films are necessary.

If any part of the urinary tract is not well demonstrated, take an additional prone film after 15 minutes. (This will be 25 minutes after the injection was started.)

Then add the film of the bladder: check this. If there is any doubt about the lower ureter or bladder, take a film after the patient has emptied the bladder.

## Immediate Post-Injection Film

A film taken immediately after injection should show the kidneys increased in density because of the contrast within the kidney tissue. Look at the shape and size of the kidneys. If either or both of the kidneys are not seen in the usual position, look everywhere in the abdomen. The kidney may have been pushed or displaced to an abnormal position, even into the pelvis.

Next, check the outline of the kidneys; make sure it is smooth. Any irregularity may indicate a scar or a mass. If you know from the plain film that there is a mass (a bulge) in one part of the kidney, see whether it is the same density as the kidney substance or remains unchanged following the injection. Failure of the mass to increase in density suggests that it is a cyst without significant circulation. If it increases in density with the rest of the kidney, a tumour is most likely.

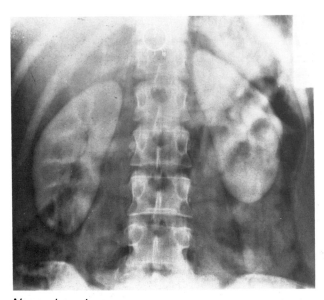

*Normal nephrogram*

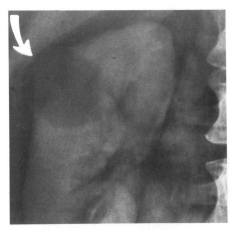

*Renal cyst*

## Ten-Minute (or Later) Radiographs

At this stage the calyces, renal pelvis, and at least part of the ureters will normally be visible. There is considerable anatomical variation in the number and shape of the renal calyces, but they are usually reasonably symmetrical on each side (see page 199). If one kidney (or both) appears to have two separated groups, upper and lower, look for an additional ureter which may join the normal ureter close to the pelvis or may remain separate and enter the bladder separately.

In the 10-minute or later film, the nephrogram should be less obvious on both sides; both kidneys should have the same density.

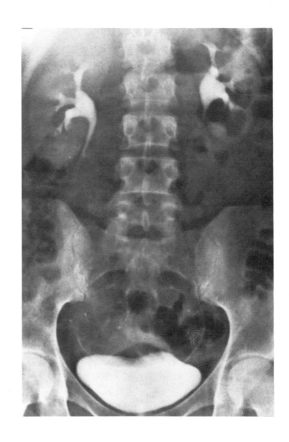

*Normal urogram 10 minutes after injection of contrast solution*

The kidneys, ureters, and bladder are all normal. Owing to peristalsis, the normal ureter is not usually filled throughout its length.

*Function*

When one kidney is denser than the other, this is due to persistence of the contrast material in the kidney (a persistent nephrogram) and suggests ureteric obstruction. It may not be possible to recognize the calyces, pelvis, or ureter on the side of the dense kidney. A film should then be taken 40 minutes later; this will usually show the ureter at the level at which it is blocked, as by a calculus.

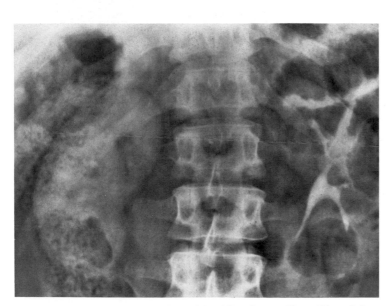

The left kidney is normal in this 10-minute film. The right kidney is dense and the calyces and pelvis are not seen.

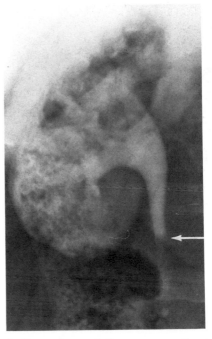

A film taken of the same patient 40 minutes later shows the calculus within the ureter. This caused the "obstructive nephrogram".

## "Missing" Kidney

If a kidney is not seen after ten minutes it must be:
(a) absent,
(b) displaced or ectopic, or
(c) non-functioning or poorly functioning.

(a) Search the abdomen for a nephrogram or any part of the calyces, renal pelvis, or ureter in the abdomen. The kidney may have been removed, destroyed, or may never have developed adequately. When this happens the other kidney is usually larger in size, but otherwise normal (compensatory hyperplasia).
(b) Displacement of a kidney is usually due to a developmental variation, but an enlarged spleen or liver or any other mass can move the kidney sideways or downwards. A large renal mass may also cause displacement.
(c) A non-functioning kidney may be due to:
   ( i) Obstruction, with or without hydronephrosis.
   ( ii) Renal tissue which may have been destroyed.
   (iii) If less than 40 ml of contrast medium has been injected, the delayed nephrogram may not be recognized, especially where there is or has been recent renal colic. Re-X-ray in 30 minutes (see previous page) or repeat the injection with an additional 20 ml of contrast and re-X-ray 10 minutes after this injection.

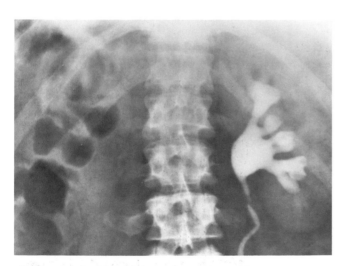

*Absent right kidney*

The left kidney is hyperplastic in compensation.

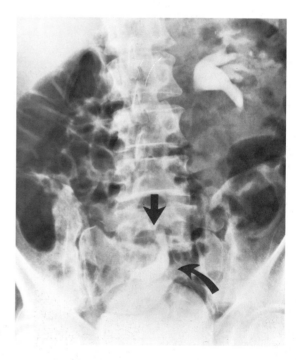

*Ectopic, low right kidney*

The renal pelvis can be seen just above the bladder. When you see this, make sure that there is no mass displacing the kidney downwards.

## Variations in Anatomy

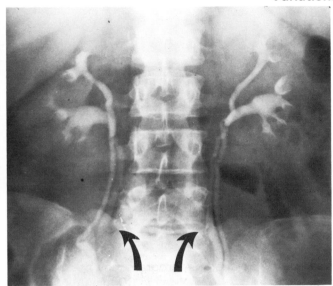

There are many anatomical variations in the kidneys and ureters, but these do not always affect renal function. The ureters may be double on both sides or on one side only. The divided ureters may join near the renal pelvis, further down in front of the sacro-iliac joints, or close to the bladder. Sometimes one ureter (always from the upper part of the kidney) joins the bladder below the usual ureteric orifice, or even drains directly into the vagina or male urethra. This is one of the causes of urinary incontinence in females. Most anatomical variations do not require treatment unless complicated by additional disease—e.g., calculi, or hydronephrosis.

*Bilateral double ureters*

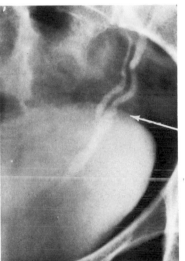

*Ureters joining close to the bladder*

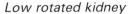

*Duplex kidney*

Sometimes the kidney is partially divided (a duplex kidney), as this left kidney. The upper ureter joins the renal pelvis.

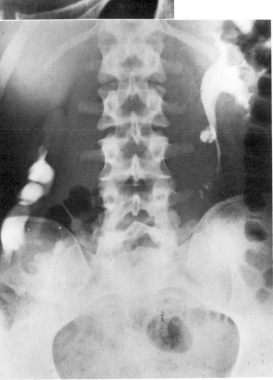

*Low rotated kidney*

The kidney may be low in the abdomen and partially rotated, as this right kidney. A film taken with the patient rotated 45° towards the rotated kidney will often show a more normal appearance. (Note the calcified lymph node overlying the left ureter.)

## Variations in Anatomy *(continued)*

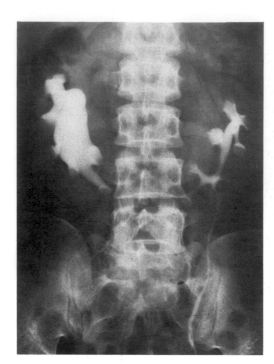

### *"Horseshoe" kidney*

The two kidneys may be joined together across the midline, nearly always at the lower poles. This is a "horsehoe" or "U" kidney. The calyces are then pointing medially or backwards instead of laterally, and the ureters come from low in the kidneys on the lateral rather than the medial side.

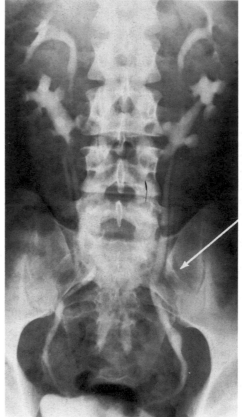

### *Duplex-horseshoe kidney*

This kidney is divided and has divided ureters. The lower part of each kidney is joined across the mid-line, so this is a duplex-horseshoe kidney, with double ureters. (The ureters join in front of the sacro-iliac joints.)

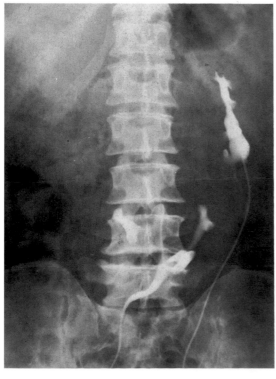

### *Crossed-ectopia*

The kidneys may both be on the same side (a condition called "crossed-ectopia"). They may be separate but are usually joined together ("fused crossed-ectopia"). One ureter is short, the other more normal in length. (In this film there are retrograde catheters, one in each ureter.) Apart from being in the wrong place and joined together, such kidneys are often rotated, which results in a rather strange urogram.

## Calyceal Patterns

*Variations in the normal calyceal patterns*

There is a very wide range of variation in the normal calyces. There are usually three major calyces, each with two minor calyces at the end. However, there may be only two major calyces and the renal pelvis may also divide into two, or there may be a single large renal pelvis with minor calyces arising directly from it. Almost any combination is possible, but all the calyces should be smooth and the "cup" at the end, surrounding the renal papilla, should be seen. If the kidney is rotated the calyces can appear "blunted", but if there is any clinical doubt turn the patient obliquely and re-X-ray.

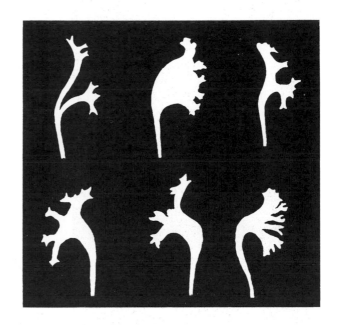

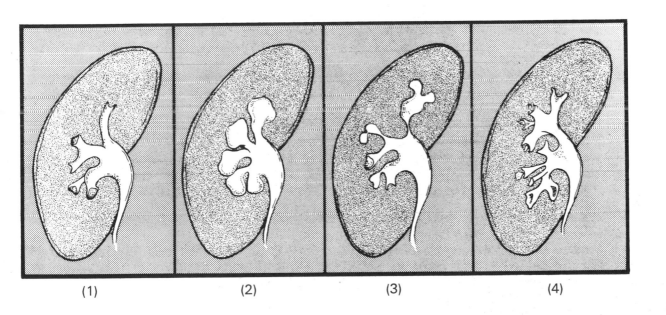

(1)    (2)    (3)    (4)

(1) *Normal renal pelvis, 3 major calyces, 4 minor calyces*
(2) *Mild back-pressure hydronephrosis*
   The "cup" has been blown out and blunted owing to ureteric obstruction.
(3) *Scarred and distorted upper pole and upper mid-pole calyces*
   These may be due to old pyelitis or perhaps renal tuberculosis.
(4) *Papillary necrosis*
   The renal papillae have separated and some of the calyceal cups are blunted (lower pole) with debris in them. Seen in sickle-cell disease, diabetes mellitus, excess acetylsalicylic acid or phenacetin usage, pyelo-nephritis, and, rarely, in hepatic cirrhosis.

## Calyceal Patterns *(continued)*

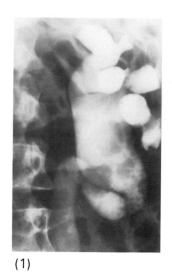

(1)

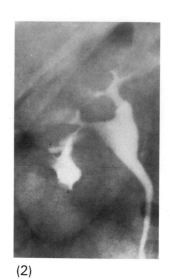

(2)

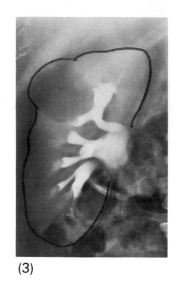

(3)

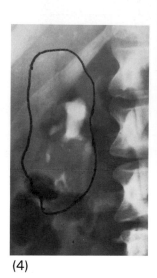

(4)

(1) Hydronephrosis and hydroureter due to obstruction of the ureter. If bilateral, usually caused by bladder outlet obstruction—e.g., enlarged prostate, urethral valves, or stricture. Renal tissue will be diminished when there is hydronephrosis. A large renal pelvis may be mistaken for hydronephrosis. Ask for a second opinion.

Normal physiological pelvic and ureteric dilatation may persist up to three months after parturition.

(2) Lower pole calyx destroyed by infection, usually tuberculosis or local recurrent pyelitis with a calculus. Other calyces normal in this case.

(3) Displaced upper pole calyces, pushed apart by a renal cyst (see page 194).

(4) Small scarred calyces, shrunken renal outline, especially lower pole. The result of chronic pyelitis and subsequent scarring. Can affect all or any of the poles of the kidney (not necessarily symmetrically if both kidneys are affected). Distinguish between fetal lobulation (no loss of renal tissue) and chronic pyelitis (irregular loss and narrowing of renal tissue). Congenital small kidneys also exist.

If the renal contour curves *inwards,* towards the distorted calyces, there must be scarring of the parenchyma from old infection, surgery, trauma, or infarct.

If there is a localized *outward* bulge in the contour, with distorted calyces, there must be a renal cyst (the most common cause, especially in older patients), a renal tumour, an abscess (pyogenic or tuberculous), or a haematoma following injury.

---

UNEXPLAINED CHANGES IN RENAL SHAPE ARE AN INDICATION TO REFER THE FILMS FOR A SPECIALIST OPINION.

## Large Kidney

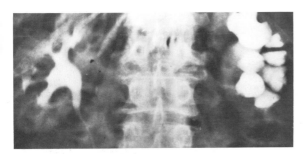

*Hydronephrosis (left)*

All the calyces are dilated.

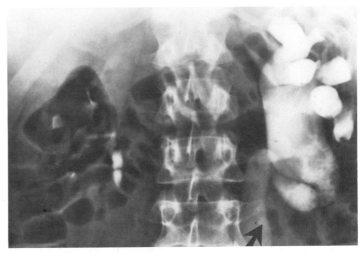

*Severe hydronephrosis (left)*

Very dilated calyces and renal pelvis. The ureter is also dilated.

*Causes of a large kidney*

(1) Hydronephrosis or pyonephrosis following blockage of the ureter from any cause (stone, stricture, etc.). This may be unilateral or bilateral, or affect half a duplex system (page 198). If bilateral, the obstruction is probably in the bladder or urethra.

(2) A renal mass causes localized enlargement. The mass may be a cyst or a tumour. If a cyst, there is no increase in density during the early post-injection phase, whereas the rest of the kidney will be dense. A tumour will have the same density as the rest of the kidney. Either a tumour or a cyst may displace the calyces as well as distorting the renal outline. If you have any doubt, refer the films for a specialist opinion.

(3) When one kidney is absent, ceases to function, or functions poorly, the other will eventually enlarge. This is compensatory hyperplasia.

(4) If both kidneys are large, without hydronephrosis, there is probably polycystic disease. The renal outline will be ill-defined, irregular but smooth.

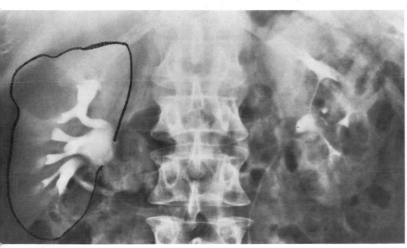

*Local renal enlargement (right) due to a cyst*

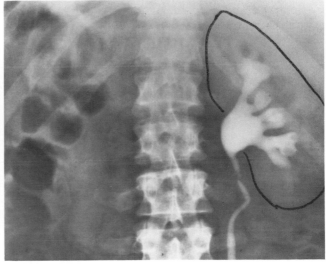

*Absent right kidney*

Hyperplasia of the left kidney.

## Small Kidney

*Causes of a small kidney*

   (1)  The kidney may never have developed completely (hypoplasia).
   (2)  Scarring following chronic infection.
   (3)  Reduced renal blood supply.
   (4)  Both kidneys may be small from the end stage of renal disease.

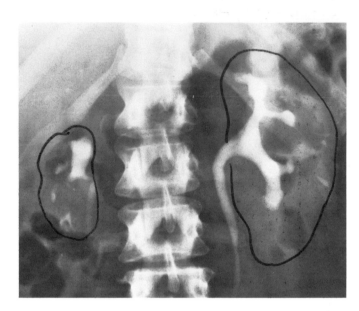

*Small right kidney due to severe repeated infection*

The left kidney is hyperplastic in compensation.

*Infection*

Small shrunken right kidney due to chronic pyelonephritis. Hydronephrosis of left kidney and hydroureter (dilated). With such hydronephrosis there is likely to be repeated infection of the left kidney associated with ureteric reflux.

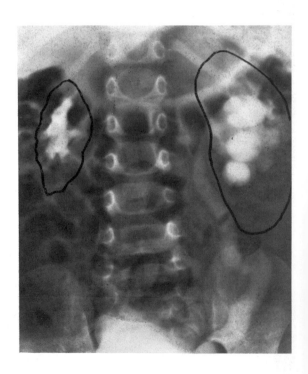

# Ureters

*Causes of dilatation of the ureters*

(1) Obstruction at any level. If one ureter is obstructed, this is probably due to a stone or a clot, or occasionally to a stricture or to a bladder tumour near the orifice. If both ureters are dilated, the cause is probably in the bladder or urethra (e.g., prostate) or valves.

(2) Reflux due to malfunction of the ureterovesical junction, from any cause with or without infection.

(3) Pregnancy. Any time after the first three months both ureters (but especially the right) undergo physiological dilatation, which may persist for up to three months after delivery.

(4) Paralysed bladder—e.g., following spinal cord injuries or meningomyelocele.

(5) Irregular dilatation, especially at the lower ends bilaterally, is usually due to schistosomiasis. If unilateral, it may be attributable to tuberculosis or the passage of a calculus.

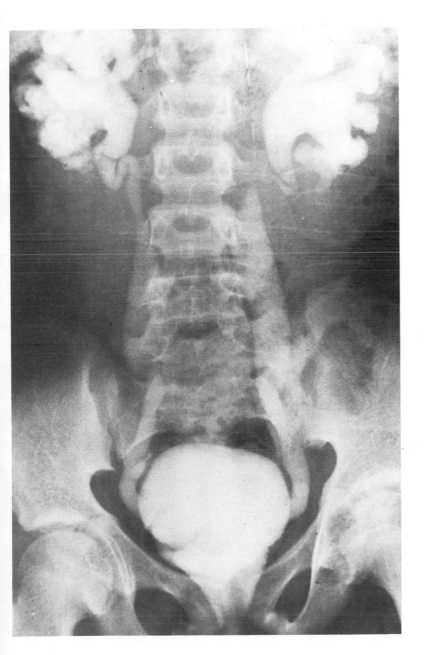

*Severe bilateral hydroureter*

The dilated ureters are due to bladder outlet obstruction. The cause varies with age. In *children* it is caused by urethral valves, phimosis, or reflux; in *adults,* by enlarged prostate, urethral stricture, or schistosomiasis.

When the kidneys and ureters are dilated like this they will usually be infected, but the real problem is the obstruction.

**Ureters** (continued)

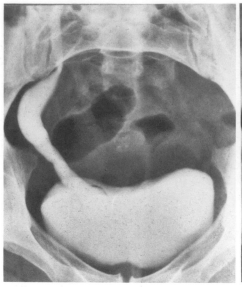

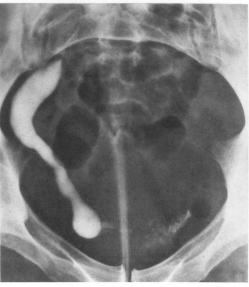

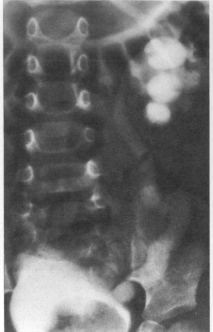

*Ureterocele*

The lower end of the ureter may herniate into the bladder and become partially obstructed. If the bladder is full, it is not easily seen. If very large it may resemble a bladder tumour and obstruct the ureter on the opposite side also.

*Displaced ureters*

Both these ureters are pushed medially. Such displacement can be due to ovarian tumours (Burkitt's lymphoma in children), fibroids, or retroperitoneal haemorrhage or tumour. When the ureters are displaced outwards (laterally) the cause is usually an aortic aneurysm or tuberculous spinal abscess. (In this patient the third and fourth lumbar vertebrae are dense because of tuberculosis.)

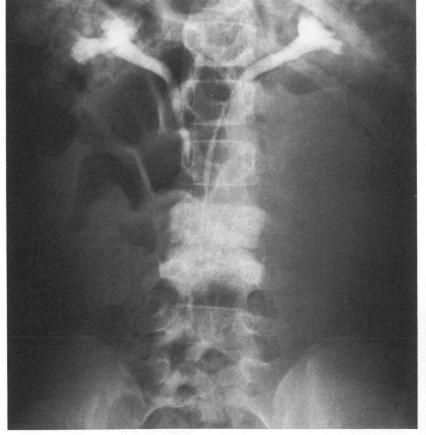

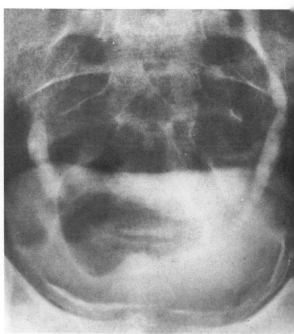

*Bilateral irregular dilated/narrowed ureters*

These are typical of schistosomiasis (note bladder calcification above the pubic symphysis). If the ureteric changes were unilateral, the cause could be tuberculosis.

## Bladder

If the bladder is to be examined following intravenous urography, look at the 20-minute film. If filling is incomplete, sit the patient up and re-X-ray after a further 20 minutes. Make sure the patient does not empty the bladder while waiting!

(1) *The large bladder may be due to:*

(a) Prostatic obstruction.
(b) Urethral obstruction (gonococcal stricture, phimosis, or carcinoma of the penis or urethral valves).
(c) Paralysis (neurogenic bladder).

(2) *The small bladder*

This follows infection, usually due to:
(a) Tuberculosis.
(b) Schistosomiasis.
(c) In rare instances, it follows pelvic irradiation or surgery associated with a spinal cord disease.

(3) *Irregular (rough) bladder outline*

(a) Rough indistinct outline of the bladder is commonly due to muscle wall hypertrophy with trabeculation or to diverticula.
(b) Chronic cystitis can also cause a very rough outline without diverticula.
(c) Neurogenic bladder is another possible cause.

(4) *Stones (calculi)*

These are often large and single and may be calcified or non-calcified. They occur in adults and children and may be multiple and/or laminated.

(5) *Calcification*

Schistosomiasis causes "eggshell" calcification, which may be thin or thick around part or all of the bladder. If calcification is in one small patch only, this is usually due to tuberculosis, but schistosomiasis or encrusted papillae may be the cause.

(6) *Local defect*

A negative defect in the cystogram is almost always due to a carcinoma of the bladder, but can be due to a non-calcified calculus or a ureterocele. A tumour is usually irregular, a calculus is usually round. If the defect is at the base of the bladder, this may be due to an enlarged prostate. There may be prostatic calcification visible below it.

(7) *Gas in the bladder*

This is usually due to a fistula between the bladder and the bowel or vagina. It can occur in severe diabetes. Do not forget the balloon of an indwelling (Foley) catheter! This is full of air also.

*Large solitary laminated bladder stone (no contrast)*

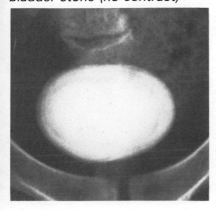

*Multiple small stones*

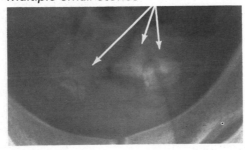

*Large bladder stone causing a negative shadow in a contrast-filled bladder*

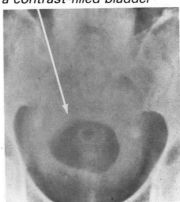

## Pressure or Distortion of the Bladder

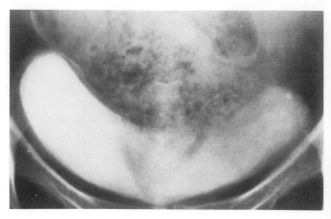

*Pressure on top of the bladder*

Usually from the uterus, ovaries, tubes or, as here, faeces in the colon.

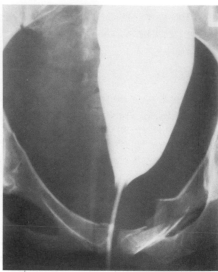

*Pelvic haematoma*

Pressure on the bladder when the pelvis is fractured usually means a pelvic haematoma. It can be unilateral or (as here) bilateral, lifting the bladder upwards.

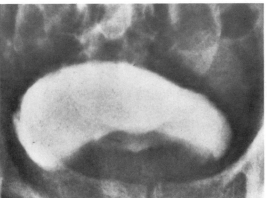

*Enlarged prostate*

Elevation of the base of the bladder usually means an enlarged prostate or prostatic abscess (provided there has been no injury).

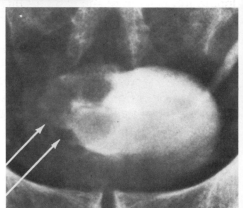

*Carcinoma of the bladder*
This is usually on one side only and often irregular in shape.

*Schistosomiasis*

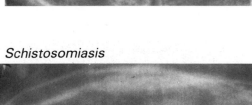

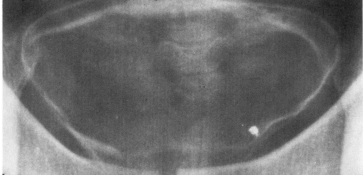

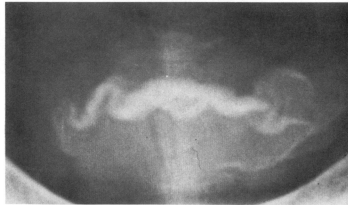

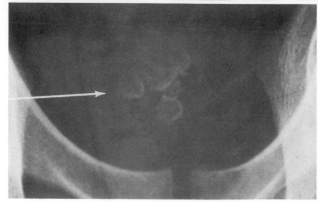

Calcification of the bladder wall is usually due to schistosomiasis. It can be thick or thin, but does NOT indicate activity. That must be determined clinically.

Local patches of calcification in the bladder wall can be due to tuberculosis or schistosomiasis or papilloma. They can resemble calculi; if in doubt, turn the patient prone and re-X-ray. Calculi will change position.

# URETHROGRAPHY

The urethra may be examined 30 minutes after intravenous urography when the bladder is filled, or by a retrograde urethrogram. A "micturating urethrogram" means that the X-ray exposure is made while the patient empties the bladder.

## Indications

After trauma, when there is blood in the urine and pelvic fracture is suspected. Do not fill the bladder through a urethral catheter: this can be dangerous. Inject contrast material and take a film of the bladder after 30 minutes. Then allow the patient to micturate if possible. The bladder may be compressed and distorted owing to blood within the pelvis (a pelvic haematoma outside the bladder wall). There may be leakage of the contrast into the pelvis because of a tear in the wall of the bladder, or through the perineum owing to urethral damage.

## Retrograde urethography

Do not do a retrograde urethrogram if there is an acute urethral infection. An ascending urethrogram can be made by injecting contrast into the urethra. Insert local anesthetic (under sterile precautions) into the urethra, and after a few minutes insert a Foley catheter until the balloon is about 1 cm from the urethral meatus. Inflate the balloon of the catheter until the patient complains of discomfort. Fill a 20-ml syringe with intravenous contrast solution, attach to the catheter and with the patient in the oblique position, inject the contrast solution. You MUST wear a lead apron and lead gloves while making this injection as the exposure must be made while the solution is being injected. If necessary, repeat the injection with the patient in the opposite oblique position. Deflate the balloon and pull out the catheter after inspecting the films.

Urethral stricture is most commonly caused by gonorrhoea but it can also result from trauma. (Check clinical history.) Catheterization of the urethra can cause significant damage. Fistulae can form into the perineum and false passages may occur alongside the stricture of the urethra. These almost always follow attempted catheterization.

## Prostatic calculi

These are seen behind or below the pubic symphysis and have no clinical significance. They do not indicate prostatic hyperplasia or urethral stricture, nor do they indicate prostatitis.

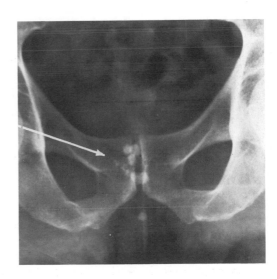

*Urethra with multiple strictures*

This urethra has multiple strictures, the most severe being in the perineal area. There is filling of the dorsal vein of the penis, which is seen when urethrography is performed following catheterization or cystoscopy. This does not require treatment. In this patient the prostatic urethra is a little dilated; perhaps the prostate has been removed.

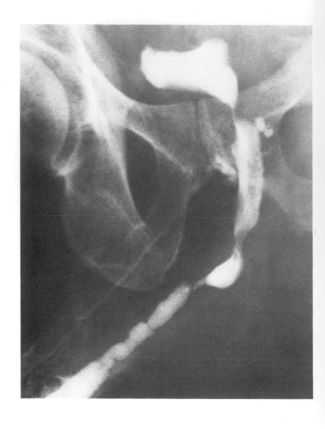

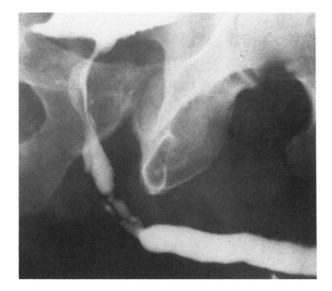

*Post-gonococcal stricture*

The stricture is in the perineal part of the urethra. There is a false passage past the stricture following catheterization. The prostatic urethra and the penile urethra are normal otherwise.

*Watering-can perineum*

Old traumatic stricture with multiple fistulae, some to the skin. The bladder is very irregular on account of cystitis.

The clinical history of local trauma will help to distinguish between the various causes of stricture.

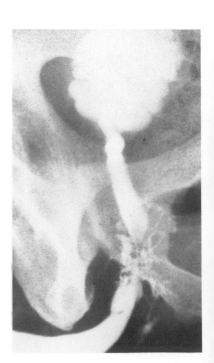

# INDEX

# INDEX

WHO publications may be obtained, direct or through booksellers, from:

ALGERIA: Entreprise nationale du Livre (ENAL), 3 bd Zirout Youcef, ALGIERS

ARGENTINA: Carlos Hirsch SRL, Florida 165, Galerías Güemes, Escritorio 453/465, BUENOS AIRES

AUSTRALIA: Hunter Publications, 58A Gipps Street, COLLINGWOOD, VIC 3066 — Australian Government Publishing Service *(Mail order sales)*, P.O. Box 84, CANBERRA A.C.T. 2601; *or over the counter from* Australian Government Publishing Service Bookshops *at*: 70 Alinga Street, CANBERRA CITY A.C.T. 2600; 294 Adelaide Street, BRISBANE, Queensland 4000; 347 Swanston Street, MELBOURNE, VIC 3000; 309 Pitt Street, SYDNEY, N.S.W. 2000; Mt Newman House, 200 St. George's Terrace, PERTH, WA 6000; Industry House, 12 Pirie Street, ADELAIDE, SA 5000; 156–162 Macquarie Street, HOBART, TAS 7000 — R. Hill & Son Ltd, 608 St. Kilda Road, MELBOURNE, VIC 3004; Lawson House, 10–12 Clark Street, CROW'S NEST, NSW 2065

AUSTRIA: Gerold & Co., Graben 31, 1011 VIENNA I

BANGLADESH: The WHO Representative, G.P.O. Box 250, DHAKA 5

BELGIUM: *For books*: Office International de Librairie s.a., avenue Marnix 30, 1050 BRUSSELS. *For periodicals and subscriptions*: Office International des Périodiques, avenue Louise 485, 1050 BRUSSELS — *Subscriptions to World Health only*: Jean de Lannoy, 202 avenue du Roi, 1060 BRUSSELS

BHUTAN: *see* India, WHO Regional Office

BOTSWANA: Botsalo Books (Pty) Ltd., P.O. Box 1532, GABORONE

BRAZIL: Centro Latinoamericano de Informação em Ciencias de Saúde (BIREME), Organização Panamericana de Saúde, Sector de Publicações, C.P. 20381 - Rua Botucatu 862, 04023 SÃO PAULO, SP

BURMA: *see* India, WHO Regional Office

CANADA: Canadian Public Health Association, 1335 Carling Avenue, Suite 210, OTTAWA, Ont. K1Z 8N8. (Tel: (613) 725-3769. Télex: 21–053–3841)

CHINA: China National Publications Import & Export Corporation, P.O. Box 88, BEIJING (PEKING)

DEMOCRATIC PEOPLE'S REPUBLIC OF KOREA: *see* India, WHO Regional Office

DENMARK: Munksgaard Export and Subscription Service, Nørre Søgade 35, 1370 COPENHAGEN K (Tel: +45 1 12 85 70)

FIJI: The WHO Representative, P.O. Box 113, SUVA

FINLAND: Akateeminen Kirjakauppa, Keskuskatu 2, 00101 HELSINKI 10

FRANCE: Librairie Arnette, 2 rue Casimir-Delavigne, 75006 PARIS

GERMAN DEMOCRATIC REPUBLIC: Buchhaus Leipzig, Postfach 140, 701 LEIPZIG

GERMANY, FEDERAL REPUBLIC OF: Govi-Verlag GmbH, Ginnheimerstrasse 20, Postfach 5360, 6236 ESCHBORN — Buchhandlung Alexander Horn, Friedrichstrasse 39, Postfach 3340, 6200 WIESBADEN

GHANA: Fides Entreprises, P.O. Box 1628, ACCRA

GREECE: G. C. Eleftheroudakis S.A., Librairie internationale, rue Nikis 4, ATHENS (T. 126)

HONG KONG: Hong Kong Government Information Services, Beaconsfield House, 6th Floor, Queen's Road, Central, VICTORIA

HUNGARY: Kultura, P.O.B. 149, BUDAPEST 62

INDIA: WHO Regional Office for South-East Asia, World Health House, Indraprastha Estate, Mahatma Gandhi Road, NEW DELHI 110002

INDONESIA: P.T. Kalman Media Pusaka, Pusat Perdagangan Senen, Block 1, 4th Floor, P.O. Box 3433/Jkt, JAKARTA

IRAN (ISLAMIC REPUBLIC OF): Iran University Press, 85 Park Avenue, P.O. Box 54/551, TEHERAN

IRELAND: TDC Publishers, 12 North Frederick Street, DUBLIN 1 (Tel: 744835–749677)

ISRAEL: Heiliger & Co., 3 Nathan Strauss Street, JERUSALEM 94227

ITALY: Edizioni Minerva Medica, Corso Bramante 83–85, 10126 TURIN; Via Lamarmora 3, 20100 MILAN; Via Spallanzani 9, 00161 ROME

JAPAN: Maruzen Co. Ltd, P.O. Box 5050, TOKYO International, 100–31

JORDAN: Jordan Book Centre Co. Ltd., University Street, P.O. Box 301 (Al-Jubeiha), AMMAN

KUWAIT: The Kuwait Bookshops Co. Ltd, Thunayan Al-Ghanem Bldg, P.O. Box 2942, KUWAIT

LAO PEOPLE'S DEMOCRATIC REPUBLIC: The WHO Programme Coordinator, P.O. Box 343, VIENTIANE

LUXEMBOURG: Librairie du Centre, 49 bd Royal, LUXEMBOURG

MALAWI: Malawi Book Service, P.O. Box 30044, Chichiti, BLANTYRE 3

MALAYSIA: The WHO Representative, Room 1004, 10th Floor, Wisma Lim Foo Yong (formerly Fitzpatrick's Building), Jalan Raja Chulan, KUALA LUMPUR 05–10; P.O. Box 2550, KUALA LUMPUR 01–02 — Parry's Book Center, 124–1 Jalan Tun Sambanthan, P.O. Box 10960, KUALA LUMPUR

MALDIVES: *see* India, WHO Regional Office

MEXICO: Librería Internacional, S.A. de C.V., av. Sonora 206, 06100-MÉXICO, D.F.

MONGOLIA: *see* India, WHO Regional Office

MOROCCO: Editions La Porte, 281 avenue Mohammed V, RABAT

NEPAL: *see* India, WHO Regional Office

NETHERLANDS: Medical Books Europe BV, Noorderwal 38, 7241 BL LOCHEM

NEW ZEALAND: New Zealand Government Printing Office, Publishing Administration, Private Bag, WELLINGTON; Walter Street, WELLINGTON; World Trade Building, Cubacade, Cuba Street, WELLINGTON. *Government Bookshops at*: Hannaford Burton Building, Rutland Street, Private Bag, AUCKLAND; 159 Hereford Street, Private Bag, CHRISTCHURCH; Alexandra Street, P.O. Box 857, HAMILTON; T & G Building, Princes Street, P.O. Box 1104, DUNEDIN — R. Hill & Son, Ltd, Ideal House, Cnr Gillies Avenue & Eden St., Newmarket, AUCKLAND 1

NORWAY: Tanum — Karl Johan A.S., P.O. Box 1177, Sentrum, N-0107 OSLO 1

PAKISTAN: Mirza Book Agency, 65 Shahrah–E–Quaid–E–Azam, P.O. Box 729, LAHORE 3

PAPUA NEW GUINEA: The WHO Representative, P.O. Box 646, KONEDOBU

PHILIPPINES: World Health Organization, Regional Office for the Western Pacific, P.O. Box 2932, MANILA

PORTUGAL: Livraria Rodrigues, 186 Rua da Ouro, LISBON 2

REPUBLIC OF KOREA: The WHO Representative, Central P.O. Box 540, SEOUL

SINGAPORE: The WHO Representative, 144 Moulmein Road, SINGAPORE 1130; Newton P.O. Box 31, SINGAPORE 9122

SOUTH AFRICA: *Contact major book stores*

SPAIN: Ministerio de Sanidad y Consumo, Centro de Publicaciones, Documentación y Biblioteca, Paseo del Prado 18, 28014 MADRID — Comercial Atheneum S.A., Consejo de Ciento 130–136, 08015 BARCELONA; General Moscardó 29, MADRID 20 — Libreria Diaz de Santos, P.O. Box 6050, 28006 MADRID; Balmes 417 y 419, 08022 BARCELONA

SRI LANKA: *see* India, WHO Regional Office

SWEDEN: *For books*: Aktiebolaget C.E. Fritzes Kungl. Hovbokhandel, Regeringsgatan 12, 103 27 STOCKHOLM. *For periodicals*: Wennergren-Williams AB, Box 30004, 104 25 STOCKHOLM

SWITZERLAND: Medizinischer Verlag Hans Huber, Länggassstrasse 76, 3012 BERN 9

THAILAND: *see* India, WHO Regional Office

UNITED KINGDOM: H.M. Stationery Office: 49 High Holborn, LONDON WCIV 6HB; 13a Castle Street, EDINBURGH EH2 3AR; 80 Chichester Street, BELFAST BT1 4JY; Brazennose Street, MANCHESTER M6O 8AS; 258 Broad Street, BIRMINGHAM B1 2HE; Southey House, Wine Street, BRISTOL BS1 2BQ. *All mail orders should be sent to*: HMSO Publications Centre, 51 Nine Elms Lane, LONDON SW8 5DR

UNITED STATES OF AMERICA: *Copies of individual publications (not subscriptions)*: WHO Publications Center USA, 49 Sheridan Avenue, ALBANY, NY 12210. *Subscription orders and correspondence concerning subscriptions should be addressed to the* World Health Organization, Distribution and Sales, 1211 GENEVA 27, Switzerland. *Publications are also available from the* United Nations Bookshop, NEW YORK, NY 10017 *(retail only)*

USSR: *For readers in the USSR requiring Russian editions*: Komsomolskij prospekt 18, Medicinskaja Kniga, MOSCOW — *For readers outside the USSR requiring Russian editions*: Kuzneckij most 18, Meždunarodnaja Kniga, MOSCOW G-200

VENEZUELA: Librería Médica Paris, Apartado 60.681, CARACAS 106

YUGOSLAVIA: Jugoslovenska Knjiga, Terazije 27/II, 11000 BELGRADE

Special terms for developing countries are obtainable on application to the WHO Representatives or WHO Regional Offices listed above or to the World Health Organization, Distribution and Sales Service, 1211 Geneva 27, Switzerland. Orders from countries where sales agents have not yet been appointed may also be sent to the Geneva address, but must be paid for in pounds sterling, US dollars, or Swiss francs. Unesco book coupons may also be used.

Prices are subject to change without notice.

C/1/87